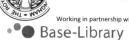

Back pain

British Society for Back Pain Research Series

Other titles in the series

Back pain: methods for clinical investigation and assessment   *edited by D. W. L. Hukins and R. C. Mulholland*

Back pain: the ageing spine   *edited by D. W. L. Hukins and M. A. Nelson*

Back pain: new approaches to rehabilitation and education   *edited by M. O. Roland and J. R. Jenner*

Back pain

Classification of syndromes

Edited by J. C. T. Fairbank and P. B. Pynsent

Manchester University Press

Manchester and New York

Distributed exclusively in the USA and Canada by St. Martin's Press

Published by Manchester University Press
Oxford Road, Manchester M13 9PL, UK
and Room 400, 175 Fifth Avenue,
New York, NY 10010, USA

Distributed exclusively in the USA and Canada
by St. Martin's Press, Inc.,
175 Fifth Avenue, New York, NY 10010, USA

British Library cataloguing in publication data
Back pain.
  1. Man. Back. Backache
  I. Fairbank, J. C. T. II. Pynsent, P. B. III. Society
for Back Pain Research
616.73

Library of Congress cataloging in publication data

Back pain: classification of syndromes / edited by J. C. T. Fairbank
  and P. B. Pynsent.
      p. cm.
    Proceedings of a meeting of the Society for Back Pain Research
held in Birmingham in March 1989, and sponsored by Butterworths
Scientific and others.
    Includes index.
    ISBN 0-7190-3272-5 (hardback)
    1. Backache – Classification – Congresses. 2. Backache – Diagnosis –
Congresses. I. Fairbank, J. C. T., 1940–   . II. Pynsent, P. B.,
1945–   . III. Society for Back Pain Research. IV. Butterworth
Scientific Limited.
    [DNLM: 1. Backache – classification – congresses. 2. Data
Interpretation, Statistical – congresses. 3. Spinal Diseases –
classification – congresses.]
  RD771.B217B32   1990
  617.5′84 – dc20
  DNLM/DLC
  for Library of Congress   90-13216
ISBN 0 7190 3272 5 *hardback*

Typeset in Hong Kong
by Best-set Typesetter Ltd

Printed in Great Britain by
Biddles Ltd., Guildford and King's Lynn

Contents

Preface

This is the fourth in a series of publications of symposia organised by the Society for Back Pain Research into various controversial topics in back pain. The classification of back pain syndromes has presented major difficulties to both clinicians and research workers in this field. This publication addresses this problem, being part of the Society's meeting held in Birmingham in March 1989. The papers are presented in two groups. The first group of papers are by specialists in various fields giving their view on the classification of patients that present to them, and some of the statistical techniques that may be used to help disentangle this problem. The second group are research papers presented to the Society. Many of these describe research in progress, and the Society provides an opportunity for discussion and the development of ideas.

It is inevitable that this common symptom is seen by a wide variety of clinicians. It is in the nature of the health-care system that various, often undefined, processes of selection of patients goes on, so that each specialist group tends to see particular subsections of patients. This should be borne in mind when trying to synthesise these different viewpoints. This book cannot and does not aim to provide the ultimate answer to the question of classification. It is hoped that it provides a useful background to clinicians and others planning research in this field. It should give clinicians in several disciplines a basis for developing their own ideas on the application of classification to the wide variety of back pain complaints that they may see in the surgery and out-patient departments.

J. C. T. Fairbank
P. B. Pynsent

Acknowledgements

The Society for Back Pain Research acknowledges with thanks the following sponsors of the meeting of Classification of Back Pain Syndromes: Butterworths Scientific, A. H. Robins Co., Merck Sharpe and Dohme, Glaxo Laboratories, Bencard and 3M Health Care.

Contributors

M. E. Barker, FRCGP, General Practitioner, The Surgery, Sheepmarket, Stamford, Lincs.

A. K. Burton, PhD, DO, Osteopath, Huddersfield Polytechnic, Huddersfield HD1 3DH.

A. Chard, MRCP(UK) Senior Registrar in Rheumatology, Addenbrookes Hospital, Cambridge.

E. N. Corlett, Scientific Advisor, Institute for Occupational Economics, Department of Production Engineering & Production Management, University Park, Nottingham NG7 2RD.

L. F. Davies, Applied Psychobiology Research Unit, School of Pharmacy, University of Bradford.

W. Deans, Mathematician, Statistical Laboratory, Department of Pure Mathematics and Mathematical Statistics, 16 Mill Lane, Cambridge CB2 1SB.

S. Eisenstein, Department of Spinal Disorders, Orthopaedic Hospital, Oswestry SY10 7AG.

F. R. Ellis, University Department of Anaesthesia, St James' Hospital, Leeds.

J. C. T. Fairbank, MD, FRCS, Consulting Orthopaedic Surgeon, Nuffield Orthopaedic Centre, Headington, Oxford OX3 7UD.

A. O. Frank, MRCP, Consulting Physician in Rheumatology and Rehabilitation, Northwick Park Hospital, Watford Road, Harrow, Middlesex HA1 3UJ.

C. J. M. Getty, FRCS, Consulting Orthopaedic Surgeon, Northern General Hospital, Sheffield.

B. R. Hammond, 137 Brighton Road, Sutton, Surrey.

B. K. Humphreys, BSc, DC, Senior Lecturer, Anglo-European College of Chiropractic Surgery, Bournemouth BH5 2DF.

D. W. L. Hukins, PhD, Department of Medical Biophysics, University of Manchester, Stopford Building, Manchester M13 9PT.
P. S. Helliwell, DM, MRCP, Senior Registrar in Rheumatology, Rheumatology Research Unit, University of Leeds, Leeds LS2 9PJ.
M. I. V. Jayson, MD, FRCP, Rheumatic Diseases Centre, Hope Hospital, Salford, Manchester M6 8HD.
M. John, MCSP, Chartered Physiotherapist, Studeley Physiotherapy Centre, 19 Station Road, Studeley B80 7HR.
J. R. Johnson, FRCS, Consulting Orthopaedic Surgeon, St Mary's Hospital, London W2.
J. R. Kirwan, BSc, MD, MRCP(UK), Consulting Senior Lecturer, Rheumatology Unit, University Department of Medicine, Bristol Royal Infirmary, Bristol BS2 8HW.
P. F. McCombe, FRACS, Consulting Orthopaedic Surgeon, Queen Elizabeth II Hospital, Brisbane, Australia.
R. S. MacDonald, MRCP(UK), MLCOM, MRO, Medical Osteopath, London College of Osteopathic Medicine, London NW1 6QH.
I. Mackintosh, Medical Physics Department, Frenchay Hospital, Bristol BS16 1LE.
C. J. Main, PhD, Consulting Clinical Psychologist, Hope Hospital, Salford M6 8HD.
B. Mathew, FRCS, Department of Neurosurgery, Royal Victoria Hospital, Belfast BT12 6BA.
W. S. Mitchell, BSc, MD, MRCP, Lecturer and Senior Registrar in Rheumatology, Hope Hospital, Salford, Manchester M6 8HD.
R. C. Mulholland, FRCS, Consulting Orthopaedic Surgeon, Harlow Wood Orthopaedic Hospital, Nottingham Road, Mansfield NG18 4TH.
V. S. Nargowala, FRCS, Consulting Orthopaedic Surgeon, Shotley Bridge General Hospital, Consett DH8 0NB.
M. A. Nelson, FRCS, Consulting Orthopaedic Surgeon, The General Infirmary at Leeds, Great George Street, Leeds LS1 3EX.
S. Nightingale, MD, MRCP, Department of Neurology, Queen Elizabeth Hospital, Edgbaston, Birmingham B15 2TH.
D. Norris, Medical Physics Department, Frenchay Hospital, Bristol BS16 1LE.
P. B. Pynsent, PhD, Director of Research, Royal Orthopaedic Hospital, Birmingham B31 2AP.
R. W. Porter, MD, FRCS, Professor of Orthopaedic Surgery, University Medical Buildings, Foresterhill, Aberdeen AB9 2ZD.
M. J. Pearcy, PhD, CEng, Lecturer in Bioengineering, Centre for Biomedical Engineering, School of Engineering and Applied Science, University of Durham, Science Laboratories, South Road, Durham DH1 3LE.
M. Roland, MRCP, MRCGP, General Practitioner, 125 Newmarket Road, Cambridge CB5 8HA.

J. A. N. Shepherd, FRCS, Consulting Orthopaedic Surgeon, Royal East Sussex Hospital, Hastings TN34 1ER.

K. H. Simpson, University Department of Anaesthesia, St James's Hospital, Leeds.

S. R. Simpson, MB, ChB, MFOM, Group Medical Advisor, Trafalgar House, 681 Mitchum Road, Croydon CR9 3AP.

F. R. Smith, Applied Psychobiology Research Unit, School of Pharmacy, University of Bradford.

B. J. Sweetman, MD, PhD, MRCP, Consulting Rheumatologist, Department of Rheumatology, Morriston Hospital, Swansea, W. Glamorgan.

A. J. Swannell, FRCP, Consulting Rheumatologist, City Hospital, Nottingham NG5 1PB.

M. Stigant, BSc, MCSP, Physiotherapy Department, Harlow Wood Orthopaedic Hospital, Nottingham Road, Mansfield NG18 4TH.

K. M. Tillotson, BSc, MIS, Huddersfield Polytechnic, Huddersfield HD1 3DH.

M. Torrens, Department of Neurosurgery, Frenchay Hospital, Bristol BS16 1LE.

J. D. G. Troup, PhD, LRCP, Royal Liverpool Hospital, Liverpool L69 3BX.

G. Waddell, Consulting Orthopaedic Surgeon, Western Infirmary, Glasgow G11 6NT.

1 *J. C. T. Fairbank and P. B. Pynsent*

Introduction – classification of syndromes of back pain

1.1 Introduction

Back pain is one of the most frequent symptoms in adults, and yet is one which has defied useful classification. Abdominal pain is also common, but it is possible to obtain an acceptably reliable diagnosis of this symptom with an accurate history, examination and a few special investigations. This diagnosis can often be validated with a laparotomy if this is indicated. Computer-aided diagnosis using this information can approach or even exceed the reliability of the most experienced clinician (de Dombal, 1984). Such precision is not yet possible with back pain.

1.2 Why classify back pain?

Diagnosis is a fundamental part of the conventional approach of Western medicine. Classification is an essential part of arriving at a diagnosis. Diagnosis forms the basis of treatment. We can only assess the results of treatment if we are sure that we are treating a particular problem or disease. We can only compare the results of one treatment with another if we are sure that we are treating the same type of patient. Audit, or quality control has become fashionable, and this can be effective only if we know what sort of treatment has been given to what sort of patient. Controlled clinical trials are only possible where patients have been carefully selected to enter those trials. Finally, and perhaps most importantly, we are unable to improve our understanding of the basic processes and the pathology of back pain without a classification of the clinical types of back pain.

Thus we see this as a most important issue which is fundamental to our understanding of this complex symptom.

1.3 **How to classify back pain**

The concept of defining syndromes of back pain is an attractive one. However, it is one which has proved extremely elusive to the many clinicians who have attempted to achieve such a classification. There is on one hand the strong clinical impression that some patients describe symptoms in a pattern which has been seen many times before but, on the other, that most patients present with such a mixture of symptoms that it defies organisation. It is possible to explain symptoms in terms of a particular pathological process or dysfunction of a particular structure, but in our view this is a temptation which should be indulged in with care until we can develop suitable criteria for classifying our patients' symptoms and signs, and until we have a better knowledge of the pathological basis of back pain.

The raw materials on which a classification can be made may divided into:

(1) History

(2) Physical signs

(3) Special investigations

(4) Response to treatment

(5) According to actual or supposed pathology

(6) A combination of any or all of these.

This book includes examples of most of these systems.

A number of syndrome classifications of the common types of back pain have recently been published. These are listed below. None of these systems are satisfying to all, but some do appreciate the difficulty in obtaining reproducible information from the patient, particularly when different cultures and medical practitioners are involved. This symposium collates a number of views on the classification of back pain syndromes. It is clear that we have some way to go before a reasonable measure of agreement can be obtained, but this book does present a number of approaches which can be explored further, and should form the basis of future research in this area.

In providing a background to this symposium, we present a number of the previous classifications of back pain, some of which have been published in previous volumes in this series.

1.4 **Some syndrome classifications of the common types of back pain**

1.4.1 *Kirkaldy-Willis & Hill (1979)*
These authors suggest five common syndromes of back pain, the names of which imply a known pathology:

    (1)   The posterior facet syndrome.

    (2)   The sacro-iliac and pyriformis syndrome.

    (3)   Herniation of the nucleus pulposus.

    (4)   Central spinal stenosis.

    (5)   Nerve entrapment in the lateral recess.

1.4.2 *Four syndromes proposed by Nelson (1986)*

These syndromes (see also Chapter 4) were proposed by Nelson on the basis of clinical features which he has found reliable in his studies of observer errors in the assessment of patients with back pain. The reliable features are:

From the history: back pain (LBP), leg pain (LP), aggravated by activity, relieved by rest, cough impulse.

From the examination: aggravated by flexion (BF), aggravated by extension(BE), limited straight leg raising (SLR), limited femoral stretch (FS), reduced reflexes.

He suggests the following syndromes:

    (1)   LBP, no LP, SLR aggravates.

    (2)   LBP, LP, BE, SLR normal.

    (3)   LBP, LP, FS.

    (4)   LBP, LP, SLR normal.

1.4.3 *Gardner* et al. *(1986)*

Gardner has described eight syndromes, which he uses in conjunction with his computer interview system (Table 1.1). Unfortunately he does not define the components of these syndromes clearly in his text.

1.4.4 *O'Brien (1984)*

O'Brien describes spinal pain in three main groups which may occur singly or in combination:

    (1)   Pain A, originates in the motion segment and its associated structures.

    (2)   Pain B, emanates from the more superficial tissues clothing the vertebral column.

    (3)   Pain C(i) and (ii) is caused by the involvement of the nerve trunks associated with the vertebral column: (i), involvement of the spinal nerve; and (ii), involvement of the sympathetic trunk.

Table 1.1   Low back pain syndrome – the Basildon system

Name of syndrome	Diagnostic category	Suggested pathology or functional disorder
1. Central myofascial pain/ tenderness	Discogenic pain	– Internal disc disruption – Disc hypermobility – Disc degeneration
	Ligament pain	– Intervertebral ligament sprain/ strain
2. Lateral myofascial pain/tenderness	Ilio-lumbar ligament pain	Primary sprain/strain
	Other ligament syndromes	– Secondary to hyper/hypo mobility of discs and other soft tissue
	Facet joint pain	– OA and degenerative changes
3. Sacro-iliac pain	Rare	– Difficult to distinguish from gluteal origin pain and referred pain from elsewhere
4. Secondary muscular pain (protective spasm reflex hypertonicity)	Muscle insertion pain	– Tennis elbow, some coccydinia, bony point pain
	Muscle belly pain	– Cramps, travel points, muscle tenderness
5. Central neurogenic pain	Central canal stenosis	– Spinal claudication – Cauda equina syndrome – Bilateral true sciatica
	Central disc protrusion	
6. Lateral neurogenic pain	Lateral recess stenosis	– True sciatica, near normal SLR
	Root canal stenosis	– True sciatica, near normal SLR
	PID	– True sciatica, marked reduction SLR
7. Mixed syndrome	One or more of the above	– Particularly after long history

Table 1.1   Cont

Name of syndrome	Diagnostic category	Suggested pathology or functional disorder
8. Radiological syndromes	Spondylolysis/listhesis	
	Infective lesions	– Abscesses
	Inflammatory lesions	– Ankylosing spondylitis
	Neoplasia	– Fracture
	Trauma	– Displacement
	Metabolic disease	– Osteoporosis, Pagets, etc.

1.4.5 *The Quebec Task Force on Spinal Disorders (1988)*
The Task Force arrived at 11 groups, which are partly based on pain patterns, partly on chronicity, partly on implied pathology, and partly on the results of investigation and treatment:

  (1)   Back pain without radiation.

  (2)   Back pain, with radiation to the proximal extremity.

  (3)   Back pain, with radiation to the distal extremity.

  (4)   Back pain, with radiation to the distal extremity, with neurological signs.

Groups 1–4 may be subdivided into those with symptom durations of:

  (a)   less than 7 days;

  (b)   7 days to 7 weeks;

  (c)   Greater than 7 weeks.

These groups in turn are divided into those who are and are not working.

  (5)   Presumptive compression of a spinal nerve root on a simple roentgenogram (i.e. spinal instability or fracture).

  (6)   Compression of a spinal nerve root confirmed by special imaging techniques.

  (7)   Spinal stenosis.

  (8)   Post-surgical status, 1–6 months after intervention.

  (9)   Post-surgical status, >6 months after intervention.

(10) Chronic pain syndrome.

(11) Other diagnoses.

1.5 Hierarchical classification

There are a large number of pathological processes which may produce back pain. To include these in a diagnostic format, one may look at the process of making a diagnosis of back pain as the penetration of a number of levels, giving a hierarchy of diagnostic precision. This approach, which may be helpful in clarifying the large, and largely anecdotal, literature on this subject, may satisfy both the 'splitters' and 'lumpers' of back pain syndromes.

The hierarchy of the known pathology of back pain is given in Chapter 2. This probably sets the gold standard for diagnosis. In practice, most clinicians see patients who fall into the subsets of 'degenerative' and 'traumatic'. Most of the other contributions concentrate on these patients, and because the link between symptoms and pathology remains remote on present knowledge, a wide variety of views are expressed. These views constitute 'syndromes'. Various methods are presented which may be applicable to the more precise definition of these syndromes. In turn these will need to be tested against more objective investigative criteria, before the most 'valid' syndromes can be established, and used in clinical trials and in studies to define the precise pathological cause of these symptoms. We believe that the technique we have described in Chapter 12 provides one weapon for establishing the precise components of syndromes. Another technique is multivariate analysis, which has been used by Waddell's group, and has been applied to rheumatoid arthitis by Kirwan, as described in Chapter 10. In turn, these syndromes can be developed into an expert system, as described by Mathew in Chapter 8, which at least provides a research tool for clinical trials and basic science investigation, and may ultimately be used in clinical practice.

1.6 Conclusion

None of these systems are satisfying to all, but some do appreciate the difficulty of obtaining reproducible information from the patient, particularly when different cultures and medical practitioners are involved.

This symposium addresses this issue, being part of the Society for Back Pain Meeting held in Birmingham in March 1989. The papers are presented in two groups. The first group of papers are by specialists in various fields giving their view on the classification of patients that present to them. The second group are papers given by members of the society which are relevant to this topic. It is inevitable that this common symptom is seen by a wide variety of clinicians, and that it is in the nature of the health care system that various, often undefined, processes of selection of patients goes on, so that each specialist group tends to see particular subsections of patients. This should be borne in mind when trying to synthesise these different viewpoints.

References

DeDombal, F. T. (1984), Computer–aided diagnosis of acute abdominal pain – the British experience, *Revue Epidemiologie et Santé Publique*, **32**, 50–56.

Gardner, A. D. H., Pursell, L. M., Murty, K. & Smith, D. G. (1986). The management of the clinical problem of spinal pain with the assistance of a microcomputer. In: *Back Pain: Methods for clinical investigation and assessment*, eds. D. W. L. Hukins & R. C. Mulholland, pp. 23–41. Manchester University Press, Manchester.

Kirkaldy-Willis, W. H., & Hill, R. J. (1979), A more precise diagnosis for low-back pain, *Spine*, **4**, 102–8.

Nelson, M.A. (1986), The identification of back pain syndromes. In: *Back Pain: Methods for clinical investigation and assessment*, eds. D. W. L. Hukins & R. C. Mulholland, pp 13–15. Manchester University Press, Manchester.

O'Brien, J. P. (1984). Mechanisms of spinal pain. In: *Textbook of Pain*, eds. P. D. Wall & R. Melzack, pp. 240–51. Churchill Livingstone, Edinburgh.

Quebec Task Force on Spinal Disorders (1987). Scientific approach to the assessment and management of activity related spinal disorders, *Spine*, **12**, 7-S, S16-S21.

Back pain – a hierarchical nosology

2.1 Introduction

Nosology[1] is the systematic classification of diseases. Back pain[2] *per se* is a symptom, it is endured at some stage of life by over 80% of the population. A taxonomy based on a symptom is an unusual approach to classification of disease. Normally disease classifications are based on the morpho-physiological systems of the body or on the pathology. The purpose of a symptom-based classification is to provide both a clinical and a research model. For this reason these models are predominantly used to classify the more elusive symptoms presenting to the clinician, such as abdominal pain and headache. Thus, in the development of a classification, we should be encompassing the complete set of all possible diseases that produce back pain as well as all the diseases which, although they may not have the symptom of back pain, are believed, by an expert, to be of spinal origin. In this chapter we develop a hierarchical classification of the diseases, compare this with other classifications and finally discover how useful the classification is in practice.

2.2 Semantics

It is important to describe what we mean by disease before we embark on the classification. A disease is a description of signs and symptoms with a known pathology and aetiology (*cf.* Scading, 1963, for a further discus-

---

[1] Not to be confused with noseology. The latter is defined in the Oxford English Dictionary as 'A study of the intellectual faculties, as manifested by the various configurations of the nose'.

[2] The terms back pain and back ache are often used synonymously. It would seem that ache is a term used more frequently by the layman, also it tends not to be used for acute severe pain.

sion). If the pathology or aetiology are unknown then the disease is often called a syndrome. Hence a disease name is really a short and convenient way to describe a pathology and aetiology with the associated signs and symptoms. In our classification, when the true cause is known we may use terms that are, strictly speaking, pathological, for example, spinal stenosis. When the 'truth' is not known, as is often the case in the degenerative diseases of the spine, then descriptions are used, causing considerable confusion with these many synonyms. Lesions associated with trauma are considered to be a disease and included in the classification. Signs or symptoms (for example, neurogenic claudication) are never included. Where possible we have tried to avoid using named structures, promoting the concept that there are two separate axes, one for disease and another defining the anatomical location of the disease.

2.3 **The hierarchy**

2.3.1 *Introduction*
This classification originated in an attempt to mimic the clinician's application of a 'surgical sieve' to the diagnostic process. The possible set of all diseases presenting to the spinal disease specialist may be split into two groups, those of the spine and those that are not. From this simple beginning, a hierarchical tree may be descended cautiously towards an explicit diagnosis (Figure 2.1).

For those diseases that are of a non-spinal origin, there seems little value in inventing some new taxonomy and thus we have just grouped all these deseases into the disease-field catagories (Figure 2.2) based on SNOMED (1987). This is in no way meant to belittle the importance of recognising these diseases clinically. For example carcinomas of the cervix, testis and

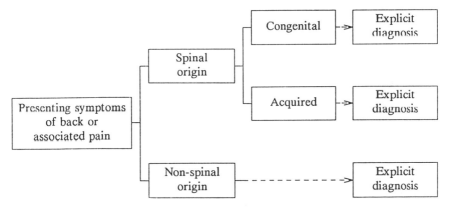

Fig. 2.1   A summary of the back pain hierarchy

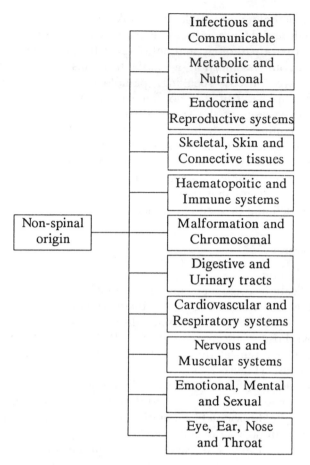

Fig. 2.2 The diseases of non-spinal origin are allocated to the SNOMED hierarchy

uterus have all been reported to present with symptoms of back pain. Following the spinal branch of the tree, the second step is to decide if the disease is congenital or acquired. The acquired diseases are split into seven catagories (Figure 2.3a) and the congenital branch is primarily split into failures of segmention and of formation (Figure 2.3b).

2.3.2 Congenital disease
The two most common congenital diseases causing back pain are scoliosis and spondylolisthesis. Scoliosis, which should probably be considered a sign, can be transformed into a disease by prefixing the cause (even though this may be idio pathic!). A full classification of scolioses is given by Bradford *et al.* (1982) and we have used this to position the disease in our

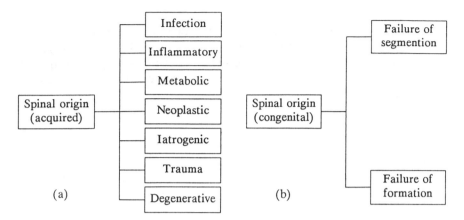

Fig. 2.3   The division of acquired and congenital diseases

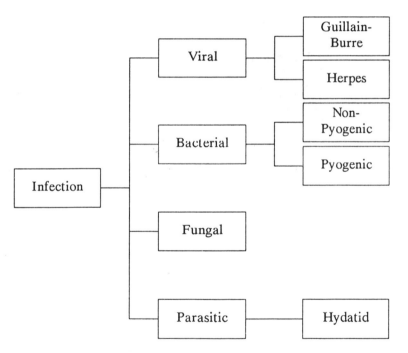

Fig. 2.4   The infection branch of the tree

tree. Congenital scoliosis may be due to either formation or segmentation failures. Similarly spondylolisthesis may be purely dysplastic or have other causes, so it will occur in several places in our classification. Achondroplastics invariably have spinal stenosis, which is often symptomatic.

2.3.3 *Infection*
Infections of the spine fall neatly into the four possible infecting agents
(Figure 2.4). The most common viral disease causing back pain is *Herpes
zoster*. Bacter-ial infections at specific sites (vertebral osteomyelitis, discitis
and sacroiliitis) are common and caused by a wide variety of organisms.
Fungal and parasitic infec-tions are rare.

2.3.4 *Inflamatory*
Rheumatoid arthritis and the seronegative inflammatory diseases are
classified in Figure 2.5. Although there is some evidence of genetic factors
and possible trau-matic trigger effects for rheumatic disease, the case for
an inflammatory branch of the tree must remain logical.

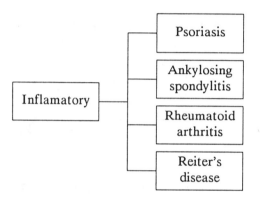

Fig. 2.5   The inflammatory branch of the tree

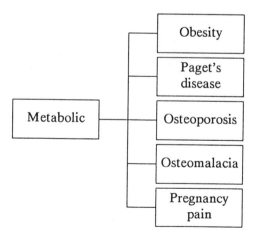

Fig. 2.6   The metabolic branch of the tree

2.3.5 *Metabolic*

The question with metabolic disease (Figure 2.6a) is whether or not these diseases are of spinal origin? This question is resolved by remembering our earlier discourse in the semantics section. Disease is really shorthand for a full description of abnormalities. For example, in the case of osteoporosis, the primary pathology may be hyperthyroidism, however the symptoms of pain, the fractures and the osteoporosis signified by radiolological results are all in the spine. These comments are also applicable to other diseases, such as osteomalacia, parathyroid disease, pituitary disease, gout and ochronosis.

Pregnancy has been placed here because of the general metabolic changes associated with it. The source of back pain during pregnancy is not clear. It may be mechanical, due to subtle metabolic changes, or both of these factors. In some cases pregnancy has been observed to relieve back pain.

2.3.6 *Neoplastic*

Neoplasms may be separated into benign and malignant (Figure 2.7). The nature of these diseases allows the tree to descend to an actual pathology (Figures 2.8 and 2.9). The incidence of these tumours has been reviewed by Dahlin & Unni (1986). Secondary neoplasms are naturally further classified by their primary site. It is worth noting that Jaffe (1958) reported that 70% of patients dying of cancer had evidence of vertebral metastases.

2.3.7 *Iatrogenic*

Iatrogenic disease may be classified into three sections as is illustrated in Figure 2.10. The incidence of mechanical factors is not known. Wiesel (1985) reports that in the USA 15% of all patients who undergo primary surgery to their back experience significant disability. Drug-induced back pain may be a result of treatments such as chemonucleolysis or a complication of treatment (e.g. heparin in pregnancy).

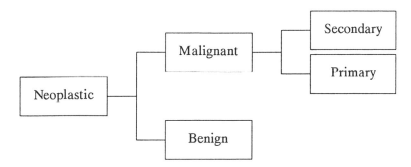

Fig. 2.7   The neoplastic branch of the tree

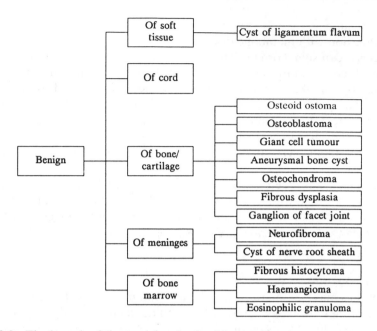

Fig. 2.8   The branch of the tree showing benign neoplasms

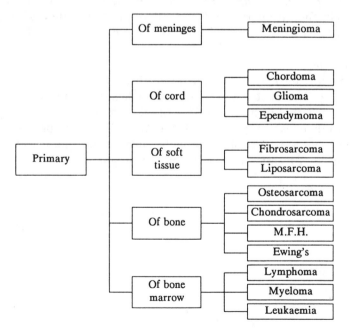

Fig. 2.9   The branch of the tree showing primary malignant neoplasms (MFH = malignant fibrous histiocytoma)

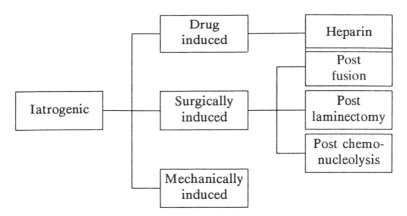

Fig. 2.10 The iatrogenic branch of the tree

2.3.8 *Trauma*

Trauma may produce damage to any of the structures of the spine (Figure 2.11a). The use of structures here is not ideal and probably the hierarchy shown in Figure 2.11b is preferable. Terms such as back strain and hyperextension syndrome occur here but what these terms mean is unclear and there is little justification, on present knowledge, in classifying beyond trauma. The nature of the trauma is part of the patient's history and does not have a place in the disease classification. In this section pathological fractures are excluded.

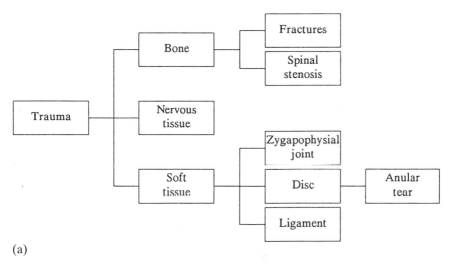

(a)

Fig. 2.11 Two possible ways (a) and (b) of classifying trauma

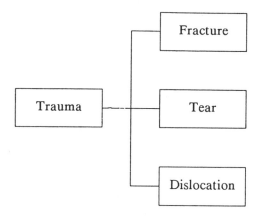

Fig. 2.11(b)

2.3.9 *Degenerative*

This includes the largest group by far of patients with back pain. As with
the traumatic diseases we propose two possible hierarchies. The taxonomy
shown in Figure 2.12a is based on the site of disease but this does not
concur with our concept of a anatomical axis. The second, more pedantic
classification (Figure 2.12b) is perhaps slightly clumsy in its approach to the
disc as a separate structure.

2.4 Comparison with other classifications

There are two widely used general classifications of diseases: SNOMED
(1987) and the International Classification of Disease (ICD-9) (1977). The
ICD-9 is basically a numbered list of diseases. This list is arranged by
pathology, anatomy, condition (e.g. pregnancy) and methods (e.g. injury)
with very little other structure, although there are hints in the 9th edition
that this may be changed in the 10th revision. The system has been extended by various specialities and of particular interest, in the case of
back pain, is the American Academy of Orthopaedic Surgeons' extension
(1986). This work takes the items of interest to the orthopaedic surgeon to
more detail by the use of additional digits. As this retains the basic ICD
code (for pragmatic reasons) it is still without structure.

SNOMED (Systematized Nomenclature of Medicine) on the other hand
is a highly structured coding system based on seven axes, each of these
being hierarchical (Figure 2.13).

There are several other diagnostic classifiations for back pain (*c.f.*
Chapter 1) but none of these attempt any form of structure. Borenstein &
Wiesel (1989) have produced a comprehensive table of diseases associated
with back pain. This is the most comprehensive catalogue that we know.

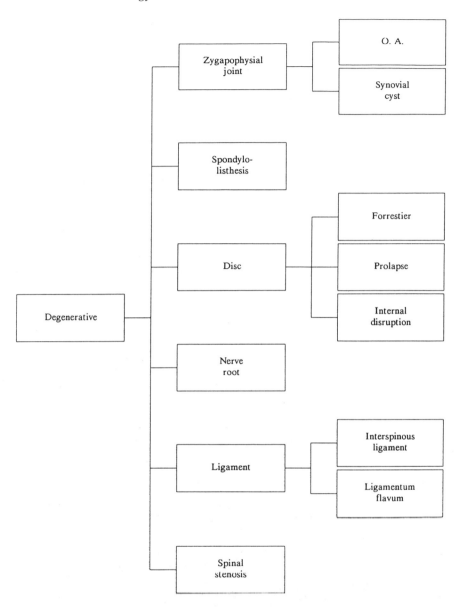

(a)

Fig. 2.12 The degenerative branch of the tree illustrating alternative classifications (a) and (b)

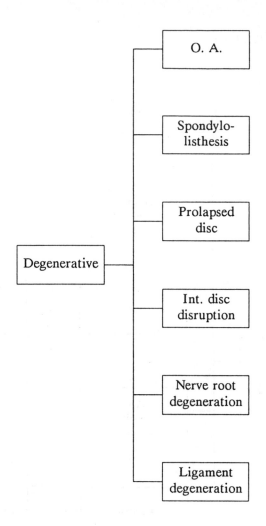

Fig. 2.12(b)

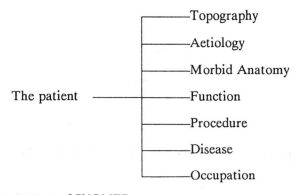

Fig. 2.13   The structure of SNOMED

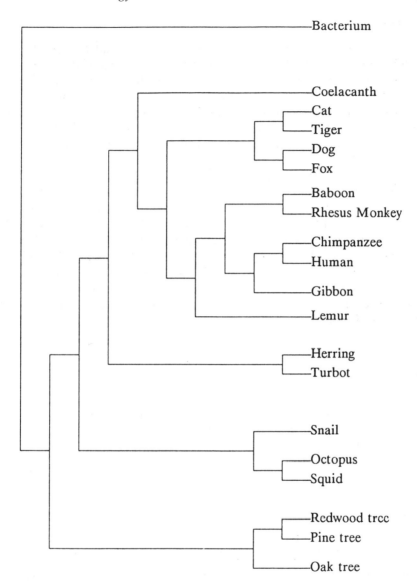

Fig. 2.14 The degenerative branch of the tree. This family tree is correct. There are 8,200, 794, 532, 637, 891, 559, 374 other ways of classifying these 20 organisms; all of them are wrong (from Dawkins, 1988)

2.5 Discussion

The hierarchical approach to classification offers some advantages. First, it enables some indication of the disease process when an exact diagnosis is not possible. Second, it allows a simple system of coding which is particularly applicable to data storage and retrieval using computers. Not only can we ask questions about the prevalence of a particular disease but also more general questions. For example, how many patients were referred to an orthopaedic department with back pain whose disease was in fact not of spinal origin?

Is this classification scheme better or worse than any other? In Dawkins' *The Blind Watchmaker* (1988), he points out, for example, that there are over 10^{20} ways of arranging 20 species in a hierarchy but there is only one that is correct (Figure 2.14). In our case there is probably no single solution. We have classified for convenience, we hope that the scheme presented is logical and educational in the sense that it highlights the difficult areas of diagnosis. It is a natural classification, constantly reducing the alternatives as we descend the tree, for this is how we like to think. The classification by its nature introduces some order into the process of diagnosing back pain.

References

American Academy of Orthopaedic Surgeons (1986), *Orthopaedic ICD.9.CM Expanded*, America Academy of Orthopaedic Surgeons, Illinois.

Borenstein, D. G. & Wiesel, S. W. (1989), *Low back pain. Medical diagnosis and comprehensive management*. W. B. Saunders, Philadelphia.

Bradford, D. S., Moe, J. H. & Winter, R. B. (1982), Scoliosis and kyphosis. In: *The Spine* (2nd Edn.), eds. R. H. Rothman & F. Simeone. W. B. Saunders, Philadelphia.

Dahlin, D.C. & Unni, K. K. (1986), *Bone Tumors*, C. C. Thomas, Springfield, Illinois.

Dawkins, R. (1988), *The Blind Watchmaker*, Penguin Books, London.

Manual of the International Classification of Diseases, Injuries and Causes of Death (1977), 9th Revision, World Health Organisation, Geneva.

Jaffe, H. L. (1958), *Tumours and tumorous conditions of the bones and joints*, Lea & Febiger, Philadelphia.

Scading, J. G. (1963), Meaning of diagnostic terms in broncho-pulmonary disease, *British Medical Journal*, **2**, 1425–30.

SNOMED, (1987), Coding manual; alphabetical index; numerical index (2nd. Edn.), College of American Pathologists, Skokie, Illinois.

Wiesel, S.W. (1985), The multiply operated lumbar spine. In: *American Acadamy of Orthopaedic Surgeons: Instructional Course Lectures*, **XXXIV**, C. V. Mosby, St. Louis, pp. 68–77. (This is quoted in Borenstein & Wiesel, 1989, p. 500.)

Discussion

Mead: Is there not a problem with hierarchial classification, that you can get stuck along one of the branches and you will not see the relationships that exist between diseases on other branches. That is, that they are not independent in the way that hierarchial classification might imply?

Pynsent (in reply): I do not wish to imply that a patient may have only one disease entity. The patient may have several pathologies, each of which would have its own end point on the tree.

Fairbank: That is an important point. Spondylolisthesis came up about ten times in the classification.

McDonald: It seems strange that in your divisions of 'spinal origin acquired' you do not have any classification for functional pathology or dysfunction, or whether it should be put in inverted commas because you do not believe in it. As there are so many people attending here who do believe in it and use it as part of what they do, it would seem appropriate to include it.

Pynsent (in reply): I do not understand what 'functional pathology' means?

McDonald: It means, as defined by Professor Barry Wyke, abnormal function in the absence of morbid anatomical change.

Pynsent (in reply): So it means physiological abnormality without anatomical change, or does it mean it is of psychogenic origin?

McDonald: Let us say, using a computer analogy, a software problem rather than a hardware problem. And there is an awful lot of software involving the back.

Pynsent (in reply): I do not accept that there is 'software', unless by this one means physiology rather than anatomy.

Frank: There are people who fulfil the criteria for hypermobility syndromes. If you put a strain through the spine of somebody whose soft tissue is much more lax than somebody who has normal soft tissues they may develop symptoms. Where would they be put in the classification, because presumably the hypermobility is hardly congenital?

Pynsent (in reply): Are you are saying that they have strained backs?

Frank: I am saying that the way the spine handles force, the same force applied upon two spines may appear the same on X-ray, but physical examination would produce pain in one person and not in another. That is one of the keys to back pain that we do not understand.

Pynsent (in reply): This I would just call biological variation.

Frank: We may be talking about biological variability. All I am saying that it does not, to my way of thinking, fit into either a 'trauma' or a 'degenerative' category.

Pynsent (in reply): I realise that, at this time, it is not necessarily possible diagnostically to distinguish the classification I have described, but at the end of the day there must be a truth. I may have the same pathology as a person who comes to your clinic, but possess a higher 'pain threshold', so I never attend your clinic. If someone comes to your clinic with pain then presumably they have something wrong somewhere. It is either of psychogenic origin, or there is some inflammation of a muscle or what ever else you might like to attribute to the term 'strain'.

Frank: Let us keep psychogenic pain out of it, because that is very rare. All I am saying is that there are people who do not fit neatly into either trauma or degenerative, and everbody sees that.

Pynsent (in reply): If you pick up something, and your back suddenly hurts, then presumably this is trauma.

Frank: Well, if that is your classification of trauma, it would not be the classification of most people here. Bending over to wash one's teeth is not exactly trauma, but I have had a number of people who have had back pain who simply bent over the wash basin to brush their teeth.

Fairbank: I think this has immediately picked up where the big trouble is in the whole of the classification. We think that there is some sort of pathological basis to the sort of patients we are talking about. We know that most of what we are talking about today is on the traumatic and degenerative part of the tree. Whether or not we include a dysfunction branch is arguable. We are not saying that this tree is the whole truth, but it does also allow us to cope with the many other causes for back ache which we all see in our practice. I think that most of the rest of this meeting is to do with degenerative and traumatic cause, but the two comments we have had, I have to say, are in the area of the art of medicine rather than its science. As long as people are using these terms, I do not really understand what they are talking about. It is important that we explore the scientific basis of these clinical observations.

3 *M. E. Barker*

A practical classification of spinal pains based on a study of patients seen in British general practice over a five-year period

3.1 Introduction

The Cochrane Committee (DHSS Working Group on Back Pain, 1979) in its summary to the Minister of Health concluded that: 'There is a profound and widespread dissatisfaction with what is at present available to help people who suffer with back pain'. The report points to the unsatisfactory treatment available and the need for research into the natural history of these disorders. It suggests, however, that it is unlikely that short term projects will be a successful means of tackling this problem. The report suggests that much of the work will have to be based on studies of the natural history of varieties of back pain, so that the time scale will be long.

3.2 Object

This survey attempted a prospective study of the incidence and natural history of backache in general practice. A classification of these disorders was then devised which should be meaningful to other general practitioners and may be of value to them in their day to day management. The classification could form a basis for clinical trials into methods of treatment of these disorders.

3.3 Method

The practice covers a small market town and its surrounding rural district extending to a radius of 5 miles. During the 5-year survey the practice size remained at about 3000 patients. Only those patients seeking a consultation specifically to complain of backache or sciatica were admitted to the survey. Backaches occurring as part of a febrile illness were excluded, as were backaches accompanied by a catalogue of other complaints.

Once a decision has been made to admit the patient to the survey a standard data sheet was completed. The information recorded included the patients name, age, sex, marital status and occupation. A careful history was taken of the present episode and of any past history of backache. The patient's description of the distribution of the pain was drawn onto a homunculus. A full examination was then performed and the findings recorded in a standardised manner.

In a survey of this kind much depends on the ability of the patient to recall past events and on the interpretation placed on these episodes by the recorder. Hirch *et al.* (1969) identified this problem and using a random sample of his original survey group re-interviewed them one year later. When the results were compared he found the reliability of the initial history to be excellent. Cobb found minimal inconsistencies when he re-interviewed a series of patients with arthritis and rheumatism where the history was taken by the same observer (Cobb *et al.*, 1956).

3.4 Results

There were 486 recorded episodes during the 5-year survey (Table 3.1). Analysis of these episodes indicated that diagnosis, treatment and prognosis could be improved by a study of the following key factors in each case:

(1)   The history of the onset of the pain.

(2)   The pattern of the pain.

(3)   The patient's perception of the quality of the pain.

(4)   The patient's previous experience of back pain.

(5)   The patient's reaction to his pain.

General practitioners may also be familiar with the patient's social and employment situation. Taking these factors into account five main groups can be identified and were labelled as:

(1)   Acute lumbago group.

(2)   Acute mechanical derangement syndrome.

(3)   Acute sciatica group.

(4)   Sacro-iliac group.

(5)   Mild sciatica group.

The features of these groups are now considered.

Table 3.1 A summary of the characteristics of the back pain syndromes (5-year study, 486 new episodes)

Syndromes	Frequency	Site of pain	Onset	Severity	Age groups	Sex ratio	Past history	Recurrence within 5 yrs
Acute lumbago	40%	L, R or central	Gradual	Variable	All ages	F > M	50%	50%
Acute mechanical derangement	20%	50% low back, 50% low back and thigh	Sudden	Severe	All ages	M = F	60%	50%
Acute sciatica	10%	Low back and leg	Variable	Severe	20–60	M = F	100%	65%
Mild sciatica	15%	Low back and leg	Gradual	Tolerable	30–60	3F = 1M	–	75%
Sacro-iliac syndrome	5%	Buttock to leg	Variable	Variable	All ages	M = F	50%	–
Unclassified	10%	–	–	–	–	–	–	–

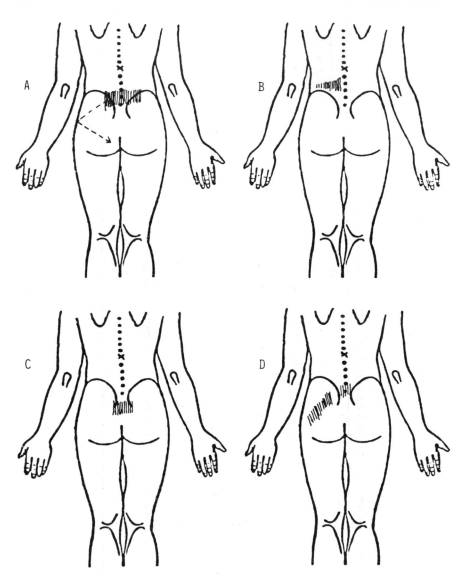

Fig. 3.1   Group 1. Acute lumbago, typical pain patterns: (a) central type of acute lumbago (in occasional cases the pain may radiate to the groin); (b) loin pain type of acute lumbago (can be left or right side); (c) sacral type of acute lumbago (d) central radiating to left or right buttock.

3.5 **Description of the groups**

3.5.1 *Acute lumbago*

This is the largest group with 40% of episodes. The patients presented with pain in the lumbar area, in the occasional case the pain radiated round to the groins or down to the buttocks (Figure 3.1). The pain developed gradually over a period of a few days. Patients of all ages were subject to this pain. In the survey the youngest was 14 and the oldest 80 years old. The maximum incidence fell in the third and fourth decades. More women than men were affected (three women: two men).

Enquiry into the past history revealed that half the patients had never had pains like this before. A quarter had had one or two previous episodes. The final quarter could detail three or more previous attacks of acute lumbago. Those patients who had presented early often had the greatest pain and the most difficulty in co-operating with the examiner. Spinal movements were severely limited as was straight leg raising. Those who presented later in the clinical course of the disorder usually had less limitation of spinal movements and straight leg raising. In no case was any motor, sensory or reflex loss found on examination. Half of the men presenting with this syndrome put their symptoms down to a recent traumatic incident or bout of heavy labouring.

The usual advice given to these patients was rest in bed for a few days with simple analgesics as required for the pain. The application of local heat and massage helped many patients. An optimistic prognosis was given and speedy resolution was usual in 1–2 weeks. No special investigations were arranged. Advice was given on posture, exercises and lifting techniques. No mention was made of possible recurrence but the follow up suggests that half of these patients can expect a recurrence whilst the other half will have no further trouble. The acute lumbago group is made unnecessarily difficult to understand because of the intrusion of many cases which do not fit the basic clinical pattern.

As many as 30% of cases appear initially to have a similar clinical picture, as detailed above, but variations in the history, examination or clinical course alert the physician to re-assess the situation.

The following problems (and possibly many more) will be seen as complications of the basic pattern:

(1) patients with spinal structural problems such as those with spina bifida occulta, suspected clinically and demonstrated radiologically;

(2) patients with pelvic tilt possible secondary to an arthritic hip or knee or an abnormality of the feet or as a result of an inequality in leg lengths;

(3) adolescents subject to acute lumbago often as a result of over vigorous exercise (Grantham, 1977);

(4) patients with 'rheumatism';

(5) patients with gynaecological or urological problems;

(6) patients who are depressed;

(7) patients who are obese;

(8) patients with medical problems such as osteoporosis, osteomalacia or spinal secondary deposits;

(9) patients with orthopaedic problems such as unsuspected spinal fracture;

(10) patients with 'clicky back' syndrome. These patients are well known to osteopaths as they respond magnificently to manipulation. These patients may be suffering from a hypermobility of the joints and from time to time get acute lumbago following a minor strain but respond quickly to manipulation until the next time;

(11) patients who are subsequently found to be suffering from backache whose problems may be elsewhere – possibly a physical problem (i.e. prodromal *Herpes zoster*) or psychological or social problems presenting in this way.

The acute lumbago syndrome is the largest group of episodes but as many as a third of the patients in this group will fall into the category of 'odd ones out' and the prognosis for these cases is that of the underlying condition. When the odd ones out are identified and excluded then the picture of acute lumbago is more easily analysed and its natural history more predictable.

In conclusion many of these episodes may be due to strained or torn ligaments and muscles in the lumbar spine, and recovery can be confidently expected provided that the patient rests, but as many as half of these cases can expect a recurrence of symptoms within 5 years.

3.5.2 *Acute mechanical derangement syndrome*

About 20% of all episodes will fall into this group. These patients present a history of pain starting suddenly, often dramatically. The pain patterns frequently encountered are shown in Figure 3.2. The patient may have stretched in bed first thing in the morning or bent over and twisted picking up a light object. In any event the patient often feels that something gives way or moves in the back. The initial movements seem to be bending, stretching or twisting movements and at some point the ligaments and

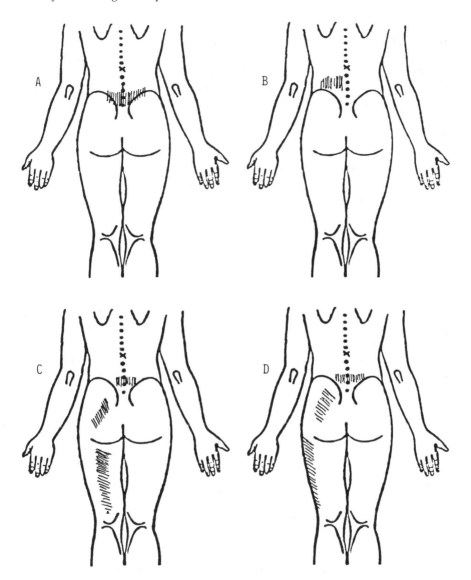

Fig. 3.2 Group 2. Acute mechanical derangement syndrome, typical pain patterns. In 50% of the cases the pain is referred to one of the legs as shown: (a) lumbar type of pain pattern; (b) loin pain pattern; (c) pain in back and posterior thigh; (d) pain in back and lateral thigh

joints become unprotected by the normal musculatory compensatory mechanisms and the unprotected back 'gives way'.

In half of the cases the pain was in the lumbar region only. In the other half the pain was felt in the back and radiated to the buttock or thigh in the posterior, lateral or anterior aspect of the leg.

All age groups can be affected with this pain but it is commonest in the 20–30 age group. Men and women are equally affected. Enquiry into the past experience of backache reveals that one third of these patients have never had this sort of trouble before, one third have had a previous episode and the remainder have had multiple attacks. Examination of the patients who present in the acute phase is often difficult. They have pain with the slightest spinal movement and can be said to be virtually 'locked'. Straight leg raising is limited and painful.

Those who are seen later in the clinical course were beginning to loosen up with improving spinal movements and straight leg raising. There was no alteration in sensation, loss of motor power or reflex changes in these patients.

A few of these patients put their troubles down to a recent episode of trauma or heavy lifting, but in the majority of cases this was not so. The usual advice for these patients was bed rest for a few days with suitable analgesia. Mobilisation was the rule after the acute pain had subsided. A simple rotary spinal manipulation appeared to speed up recovery in this group of patients if performed after the acute pain had subsided (Bourdillon, 1970).

No special investigation was advised. A rapid return to work was often achieved. Advice was given on posture, exercise and lifting techniques. An optimistic prognosis was always given despite the fact that follow up has shown that 50% of these patients will have a recurrence within 5 years.

A careful reappraisal of patients in this group shows that the category of 'odd ones out' does not apply to any great extent, only about 15–20% of these patients might have been so classified. This group mainly involves normal people with normal backs, who make an unprotected movement.

3.5.3 *Acute sciatica*

Ten percent of all episodes fall into this group. Most of these patients were seen initially at home, in bed, in severe pain. The pain affected the back, buttock, posterior , thigh and calf. In the occasional patient the pain affected the back and anterior thigh. The pain encountered is shown in Figure 3.3.

The quality of pain experienced by these patients was different. They described the pain as severe, often unremitting, deep in the back and leg, not at all like the referred pains described in the previous groups.

Men and women were equally affected by these pains, and age range in

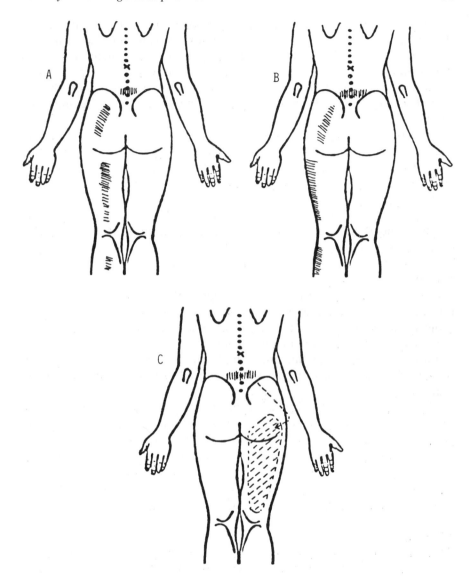

Fig. 3.3 Group 3. Acute sciatica, typical pain patterns: (a) pain in the back, posterior thigh and calf with occasional radiation to the foot; (b) pain in back and lateral thigh and calf; (c) pain in back and anterior thigh.

the survey was 20–60 years old. All these patients had a history of one, two or three attacks of backache previously.

Examination of these patients was often difficult as they were in bed, in pain, and unable to co-operate, but in all cases spinal movements and straight leg raising were severely limited. In one third of these patients no alteration in motor power, sensation or reflexes was found. Two thirds of these patients had demonstrable neurological deficits, usually a demonstrable alteration in sensation, motor power or reflexes, but two patients in the survey complained that their leg not only felt weak but was numb and cold. This might suggest that the autonomic nerve supply to the limb was affected.

All patients in this group were treated conservatively with rest in bed and suitable analgesia. When the pain was very severe the author injected local anaesthetic very deeply into the most tender areas of the back with gratifying relief of pain and surprisingly in two cases instant improvement in straight leg raising.

Despite conservative treatment for up to 2 weeks, patients often relapsed and there seemed no way to predict or prevent these painful recurrences. Full investigation was undertaken in many of these patients but often investigation was undertaken to boost morale, pass time and reassure the author and patient.

Upon the failure of conservative treatment a third of this group required referral for out-patient and in-patient treatment. These patients were subjected to prolonged bed rest, traction, epidural anaesthesia and two of the patients have now had a laminectomy.

Two other patients in this group had spinal secondaries causing their sciatica, fortunately this diagnosis was clinically suspected and investigation was initiated at an early stage.

These patients are probably suffering from disc prolapse. In two thirds of these patients conservative treatment was sufficient to achieve resolution, but one third were referred for hospital treatment. Long term follow up of these patients has shown that a third will recover despite relapses usually within a year. Two thirds will have recurrent back troubles and a few of these patients will have permanent neurological damage like a numb toe, numb patch on the calf, a lost ankle jerk or a weak dorsi-flexor of the foot.

3.5.4 *Mild sciatica*

About 15% of episodes were in this group. Usually these patients reported to the surgery for the initial consultation. The diagnosis was made on the patient's description of pain, often insidious in onset, often intermittent, often affected by posture, usually affecting the low back, buttock and leg, associated with almost full or only slightly restricted spinal movements and full or nearly full straight leg raising. In no cases were there motor, sensory or reflex deficits demonstrable.

Half of the patients in this group could recount an episode of major trauma which had initially set off their troubles often months before. Some of these patients had concluded that they had 'sciatica', but some thought it was 'rheumatism', to do with the 'circulation', a 'trapped nerve' or 'arthritis' that was causing the trouble. Some patients had not associated the back with the leg pains. These patients were slow to seek a consultation often having suffered the pains on and off for weeks or months before consulting. Most were happy to accept a diagnosis of 'mild sciatica'. Mobilisation was encouraged from the outset. Simple oral analgesia was advised as required. The patients were advised on posture and lifting techniques.

Three quarters of this group were found at follow up not to have improved. They continued to have recurrences of back and leg pain but seldom sought advice, apparently preferring to rest and treat themselves during the acute phases and put up with this recurrent back problem. To find so many chronic sufferers in this group was disturbing.

These symptoms and signs were of little interest to the practitioner and the patients apparently only consulted for reassurance that this was a benign condition assuming, possibly quite rightly, that not much could be done to help them. Mild sciatica is usually a female complaint (three women: one man).

It appears to be a chronic, intermittent condition and often (30%) stems from previous major spinal injuries. Most of these patients had accepted that they now had a 'weakness' and would be troubled with this regularly. In this group were also patients who seemed to be using this particular chronic pain pattern as a device to fall back on in times of personal stress.

3.5.5 *Sacro-iliac syndrome*

This is a small group, 5% of the total. Analysis of the features of this group is therefore not easy nor yet wholly meaningful.

All age groups were present in this group with males and females equally affected. The classification of episodes into this group rests in the pain pattern demonstrated by the patient. The pain, often severe, was felt deep in the buttock and not the back, with a radiating pain down the posterior or lateral thigh. Two patients complained of paraesthesias in the foot as well as the leg pain. Spinal movements were not restricted or painful. Straight leg raising was painful and restricted. There was no alteration in sensation, motor power or reflexes. Deep palpation over the sacroiliac joint always produced a deep tenderness.

The acute pain usually subsided after 1–2 weeks and most patients recovered in 6 weeks.

The usual prescription was bed rest and suitable analgesia. After the acute pain had subsided an attempt was made to manipulate the sacroiliac joint. In a third of cases this was successful and rapid relief of pain then occurred.

A quarter of the women in this group were pregnant at the time of onset of symptoms whilst a quarter of the men had developed the pain after a back injury.

3.6 Discussion

This survey records experience of patients with back and leg pains in a single general practice over a 5-year spell. Ninety-five per cent of all recorded episodes fell into these five groups, the residual cases were found impossible to classify as their pains fitted none of these clinical pictures, but the numbers involved were too small for meaningful analysis. No real attempt was made to set this classification on a formal pathological basis, it seemed more useful to classify patients by clinical picture.

It appears that people have either good or bad backs. If a patient has a good back it does not rule out the fact that he may whilst over-stretching develop an acute mechanical derangement of his back, he may strain muscles and ligaments and develop an acute lumbago, but the prognosis for him will be good. Bad backs are not so common. They may be the result of a growth disorder in childhood or adolescence, an injury, a heavy occupation, or a medical, gynaecological, urological or orthopaedic disorder.

These problems will require to be delineated and treated and the prognosis will depend on the underlying condition. The natural progression is towards resolution with a stable back in patients with 'good' backs. The picture is confused by those with 'bad' backs who although outnumbered 4:1 demand more of our attention and have a less certain prognosis.

About 10% of patients had disc prolapse. These patients were difficult to manage. Despite every effort to manage them at home a third had specialist referral. From the patients point of view, many weeks spent in bed seemed to produce only slow improvement and did not insure against subsequent painful relapses. Morale was difficult to sustain so that a second opinion often became inevitable. Unfortunately it became clear in this survey that hospital referral was not always on clinical grounds but was more often determined by the patient's demands. Nevertheless, two thirds of the patients with disc prolapse were treated conservatively at home and recovered albeit with residual aches and pains. As yet we have no way of determining which patients should or should not have urgent hospital treatment.

3.7 Conclusion

Throughout a survey of this nature one is faced with the variable and unpredictable reaction patients have to their pain. It is a clinical challenge to the general practitioner to evaluate what is psyche and what is soma in this field. On the one side the patient with the full-blown disc prolapse who soldiers on, on the other side the patient with mild back strain who spends months off work, demands full investigation and has every conceivable treatment.

Serious diseases like tuberculosis, arthritis and metabolic bone disease can produce similar pains; the practitioner must be constantly on his guard for these major disorders. The survey shows that fortunately only 1–2% of these patients did have serious underlying pathology and those who did were soon correctly diagnosed.

The value of investigation has not been studied in this survey because of the small numbers involved. Often investigations have been employed as morale boosters. A handful of X-rays and blood counts have proved valuable in diagnosis, many more have been excellent negative evidence, but the vast majority of patients had no investigations performed on them.

The management of this group of conditions will one day be placed on a sound anatomical basis but in the meantime general practitioners will continue to treat over 90% of these patients within their own practices. The Cochrane Comittee has recommended closer co-operation between the medical profession and heterodox practitioners in this field to establish a common ground and organise clinical joint trials. As yet very little has been done to evaluate the types of treatment made available by heterodox practitioners. Many general practitioners are interested in osteopathic and chiropractic techniques and are keen to learn how to apply them. In this survey possibly 50% of the patients could have been helped by manual therapy.

Resources in General Practice are at present limited to bed rest, simple analgesics and local anaesthetic injections. Corsets, traction and epidural anaesthesia are not readily available. Open access to physiotherapy and an increased availibility of epidural anaesthesia would be helpful in dealing with these problems. Meanwhile the average general practitioner will deal with two cases of lumbago or sciatica every week, and most will be offered conservative treatment.

Acknowledgement

I should like to acknowledge the assistance I have received from my secretary, Mrs S. A. Dwyer.

References

Bourdillon, W. (1970), *Spinal Manipulation*, Heinemann, London.
Cobb, S., Thompson, D. J., Rosenbaum, J., Warren, J. E., & Merchant, W. R.

(1956), The measurement and prevalence of arthritis and rheumatism from interview data, *Journal of Chronic Disease*, **3**, 134.

Grantham, V. A. (1977), Backache in boys – a new problem? *Practitioner*, 218– 26.

Hirch, C., Jonsson B., & Lewin, T. (1969), Low back symptoms in a Swedish female population, *Clinical Orthopaedics and Related Research*, No. 63.

The Cochrane Report (1979), *Working group on low back pain*, DHSS HMSO, London.

Discussion

Fairbank: In a population survey that I was involved in, it was interesting to note that only a third of people who said they had backache actually consulted with their GP. It is important that we see the context of the patients we are talking about. Each specialist is likely to have a different view on this.

Fairbank, J. C. T. (1986), The incidence of back pain in Britain. In: *Back pain: methods for clinical investigation and assessment*, D. W. L. Hukins & R. C. Mulholland (eds.), Manchester University Press, Manchester, pp. 1– 12.

Nargolwala: How do you know that there were sacro-iliac cases in 5% of the patients you mentioned?

Barker (in reply): Really only because of the pattern of the pain that the patient was giving you. He can always tell you where the pain is. The patterns I have put on the board are an amalgamation of lots of patients who usually fall into distinct patterns. The patients will say: 'The pain is quite severe just there', and it radiates down the leg. I think that really you have to take the patient's word for it. If you do a rotary manipulation on a lot of these patients, you will hear a clunk, and they will get off the bed and say: 'Thank you very much, I feel better'. This is the truth. If you happen to be pregnant, I can almost guarantee that I can do this for you.

Mulholland: The central pain patterns which you describe as acute lumbago and a mechanical derangement are very similar. Do you think, therefore, that injury and trauma is in fact producing your lumbago and, secondly, when you describe trauma are you really talking about significant trauma or what I would call the 'normal activities of life'.

Barker (in reply): At one point I was describing significant trauma and that was in the case of the mild sciatica syndrome where, at some point in the past, they have suffered major trauma. With the two first groups, the acute lumbago group where the onset is gradual, and the acute mechanical group where the onset seems to be quite sudden, the sorts of traumas that we were talking about are bending over and cleaning your teeth or sitting for a long period in a car. These are the sort of traumas that people go through 100 times a day in normal living.

The classification of back pain syndromes by reliable signs

4.1 Introduction

The management of back pain presents major difficulties due to the lack of an agreed classification. Historically back pain classifications have included a mixture of anatomical and pathological groups often comprising conditions which may or may not be symptomatic.

The traditional surgical sieve classified back pain as:

Congenital
Acquired
Infection
Inflammation
Neoplasm
Vascular
Miscellaneous.

Waddell suggested a division into mechanical and pathological, the latter group including infections, tumours, etc. (Waddell, 1982).

In order to clarify the present confusion, the author has proposed the following classification:

(1)   Clinical syndrome.

(2)   Anatomical origin of pain.

(3)   Radiological/pathological abnormality.

(4)   Function impairment.

(5)   Psycho-socio-economic influences.

4.2 Observer error

The presence of observer error in all clinical studies has been well documented (Gill *et al.*, 1973). These studies show that, in areas as diverse as X-ray reporting (Cochrane *et al.*, 1952) and breast lump grading (Yorkshire Breast Cancer Group, 1977), errors between individual clinicians and the variability of one clinician's observations must always be recognised. In 1979 the author conducted a study of back pain assessment and found that the more choice a clinician has in grading an observation the greater the resultant inter-observer error (Nelson *et al.*, 1979). For example in the measurement of SLR, if the clinician attempts to measure it precisely by means of a goniometer he introduces a very high level of error. However, if he limits the choices to normal, restricted and very restricted, there is a good agreement. It was on the basis of these studies that the following conclusions are based.

The proposed clinical syndromes are based upon reliable and reproducible features of the history and examination.

4.3 Reliable and reproducible features of back pain

4.3.1 *History*

(1) Back pain felt in mid-line in lumbar region radiating transversely to the sacro-iliac region (BP1–5).

(2) Leg pain (including buttocks) radiating in a nerve root distribution i.e. L3, L4 into front of thighs to knee, L5, S1 below the knee (LP1–3).

(3) Pain aggravated by activity.

(4) Pain aggravated by rest.

(5) Pain increased by cough impulse (CI).

4.3.2 *Examination*

(1) Pain aggravated by flexion (FLEX) (Figure 4.1).

(2) Pain aggravated by extension (EXT) (Figure 4.2).

(3) Pain aggravated by straight leg raise (SLR) (Figure 4.3).

(4) Pain aggravated by femoral stretch test (FS) (Figure 4.4).

(5) Diminished or absent knee or ankle reflex (REFL).

4.4 Proposed syndromes (based on history and examination)

The following reliable features of history and examination are used to define five syndromes of back pain, three syndromes of back and leg pain, and one syndrome of leg pain alone. The features of each of these syndromes are listed in Table 4.1.

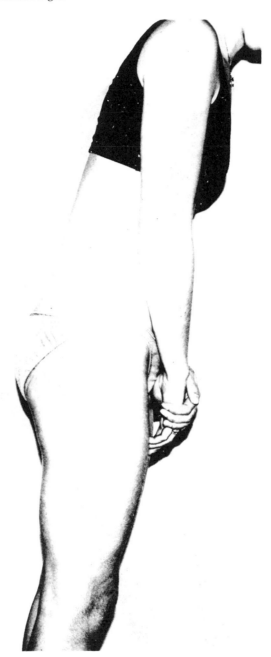

Fig. 4.1 Measurement of flexion (FLEX)

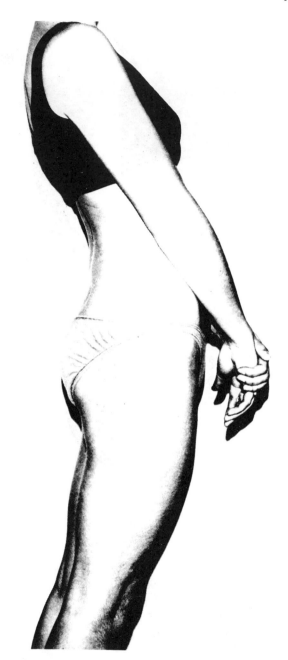

Fig. 4.2 Measurement of extension (EXT)

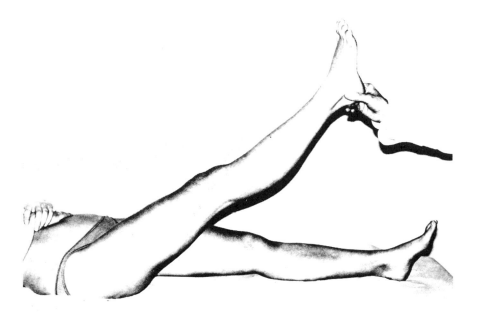

Fig. 4.3   Measurement of straight leg raise (SLR)

Table 4.1   A summary of the clinical features of the nine syndromes

Name	FLEX	EXT	CI	SLR	FS	REFL
Back pain:						
BP1	−	−	−	−	−	−
BP2	+	−	−	−	−	−
BP3	−	+	−	−	−	−
BP4	+	+	−	−	−	−
BP5	+	−	+	+	−	−
Back + leg pain:						
BP/LP1	+	−	+	+	−	±
BP/LP2	+	−	I	+	+	−
BP/LP3	−	+	+	−	+	±
Leg pain:						
LP1	+	+	+	−	±	±

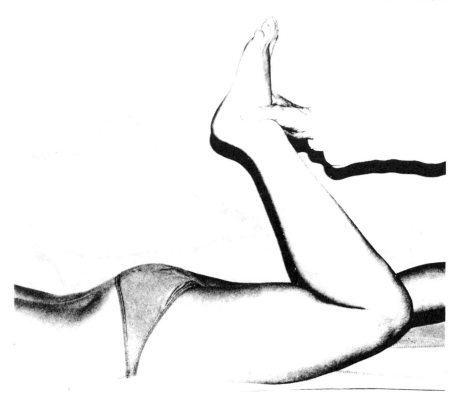

Fig. 4.4   Femoral stretch test (FS)

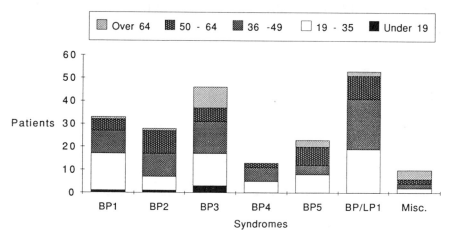

Fig. 4.5   Age distribution of the group. Others represents: two BP/LP2, two BP/LP3 and one LP

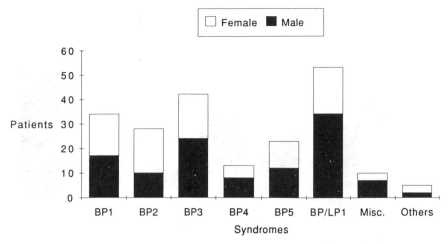

Fig. 4.6 Sex distribution of the patients. Others represents: two BP/LP2, two BP/LP3 and one LP

4.5 Clinical material

208 consecutive patients referred to a back pain clinic have been evaluated according to the syndromes described above. The incidence, treatment and results are presented. The miscellaneous group consisted of ten patients, comprising one Scheuerman's, one ankylosed hip, three O.A. hips, one old L1/L2 fracture, one ankylosing spondylitis, one osteoporosis, one Paget's and one old spinal fusion. The treatment of this group was diverse and not relevant to this chapter.

4.6 Results

The patients were assessed on the basis of reliable features of the history and examination. The numbers of patients in each group, and their age and sex distribution are summarised in Figures 4.5 and 4.6, and the treatments used in Figure 4.7.

4.7 Discussion

The art and science of modern medicine is based on the establishment of a clinical diagnosis. This began with the accurate observation of disease processes and recording the history and physical findings.

In time a wide range of conditions were recorded and identified by descriptive names, e.g. sciatica, lumbago, fibrositis.

With the advent of X-rays and blood tests more objective information

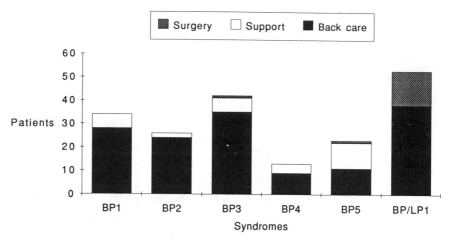

Fig. 4.7 Distribution of treatments given to the group. Back care included exercise and weight loss advice

was obtained. Recently modern investigations have permitted the recognition of conditions such as disc prolapse, spinal stenosis, etc. Nevertheless many clinical presentations are still only at the stage of clinical description without any objective confirmation.

This is true in many other medical specialities, such as dermatology and rheumatology, in which clinical presentations are labelled by descriptive terms only, without further objective evidence, e.g. erythema nodosum, synovitis, etc.

With the development of more sophisticated investigations, objective information will be added to these labels but for the time being they are all we have to go on in our recognition and management. The author suggests that in the present state of our understanding of back pain, a classification based on reliable clinical findings permits a more rational approach to management (Nelson, 1986). It is suggested that this approach to the clinical evaluation of back pain permits:

(1) a more accurate evaluation at the stage of clinical description without any objective confirmation;

(2) the accurate comparison of the results of different methods of treatment.

References

Cochrane, A. L. & Garland, L. H. (1952), Observer error in the interpretation of chest films; an international investigation, *Lancet*, **ii**, 505.

Gill, P. W., Leaper, D. J., Guillou, P. J., Staniland, J. R., Horrocks, J. C. & de

Dombal, F. T. (1973), Observer variation in clinical diagnosis. A computer-aided assessment of its magnitude and importance in 522 patients with abdominal pain, *Methodile Informazion Medizin*, **12**, 108–13.

Nelson, M. A. (1986), The identification of back pain. In: *Back Pain*, eds. D. W. L. Hukins & R. C. Mulholland, pp. 13–15. Manchester University Press, Manchester.

Nelson, M. A., Allen, P., Clamp, S. E. & de Dombal, F. T. (1979), Reliability and reproducibility of clinical findings in low back pain, *Spine*, **4**, 97–101.

Yorkshire Breast Cancer Group. (1977), Observer variation in recording clinical data from women presenting with breast lesions, *British Medical Journal*, **2**, 1196–9.

Waddell, G. (1982), An approach to back pain, *Journal of Hospital Medicine*, **28**, 187–219.

Discussion

Dowling: One of the problems I have found in clinically examining patients is that there is a variation in examining the same patient at different times. Have you considered this in your classification? This is based on whether the pain was induced on bending forwards or backwards. If you really force extension you can produce pain in a lot of people.

Nelson (in reply): In answer to your first question, I think you are absolutely right. Of course we are dealing with a symptom that gets better, and one of the difficulties is that when one sees patients again to examine them they are different. That is the nature of the symptom and of course this is why, as we are all familiar, one has to be so very critical about any form of treatment, because in fact one is dealing with a problem that gets better for most patients.

As far as the degree of bending is concerned, clearly this has to be thought about, and that is why I was trying very hard not to get tied down to measuring the distance to the ground and so on, because there is such variation. Straight leg raising is a wonderful example. I am sure if we took a patient and we asked half a dozen doctors here to do a straight leg raising test, some will stop as soon as they get pain but others will go on and on. There is no point at which we all agree that we should stop with a straight leg raising test and measure it. This could condemn the whole of clinical examination. Having said that, I think clinical examination still is the most reliable feature amongst many unreliable ones.

I am very concerned about the people who rely so much on investigations, because as surgeons we have very dangerous tools in our hands. I think we make mistakes in our diagnosis. When I see patients for a second, third or fourth opinion after having had one or two operations, clearly one had to question very much the reason for that first operation. Neurosurgeons, and I do not know whether there are any here, are still using disc surgery for back pain alone, which I hope most of us would find most amazing. But they still do it, and we have a wide problem of communication across the whole area of this subject.

Kirwan: Any classification depends greatly on the data on which it is based. Could you tell us a little bit about the 200 patients. Where do they come from?

Nelson (in reply): They were patients referred to a back pain clinic from general practitioners, from my colleagues in the hospital, and from other colleagues outside the hospital. They are highly selected but do not in any way represent back pain across the board. As we have heard from Dr Barker, I am not even sure that even his patients are representative of the whole problem. We do not have the sort of reliable database that the computer buffs would require. I accept your criticism.

MacDonald: I am trying to decide whether you are a 'splitter' or a 'lumper'. You started off by saying that you always access five items and that you would include the patient's social and economic function. You say that you assess those five things, you then spend the rest of the time classifying just one.

Nelson (in reply): Well, this is the talk we were doing today.

Dr McDonald: Well no. I think that part of the classification is the other four.

Nelson (in reply): Well of course, if we consider most patients with back and leg pain, often I can identify the site of pathology. I cannot do this with most patients with back pain.

The McKenzie classification of back pain syndromes

5.1 An overview of a physiotherapy classification

This chapter sets out to provide a comprehensive overview of the McKenzie classification of back pain – other notable schools of mobilisation or manipulation do not readily lend themselves to a structured classification.

5.2 McKenzie system of mechanical diagnosis and therapy of the lumbar spine

Robin McKenzie, a New Zealand physiotherapist, developed a technique of assessing and treating patients based on their response to repeated movements. The response of the patient to movement allows classification into one of three mechanical back pain syndromes (or diagnostic categories):

Postural syndrome
Dysfunctional syndrome
Derangement syndrome.

McKenzie based his classification of back pain syndromes on:

(1) the patient's history;

(2) the behaviour of the symptoms during everyday activities;

(3) the physical signs present on examination;

(4) the behaviour of the patient's symptoms during a standardised series of repeated lumbar movements.

There have been several papers outlining the benefits or effectiveness of McKenzie's system of treatment when compared with other forms of conservative therapy. Nwuga & Nwuga (1985) and Ponte *et al.* (1984) compared McKenzie's and the Williams protocols. Both showed significantly greater improvement in the McKenzie group. Dimaggio & Mooney (1987, a and b) used a total of 137 patients in a comparison of the McKenzie protocol, Cotterell 90/90 back traction, and back school. Patients were assessed on a visual analogue pain scale, patient pain drawings and a functional questionaire. The McKenzie group achieved a 97% success rate, 90/90 traction 50%, and back school a 38% sucess rate. These papers have taken a look at a very specific population of patients, usually derangements, and therefore the effectiveness of the total system has never been tested. Dimaggio and Mooney (1987, a and b) discuss the 'lumbar syndrome'. They define the lumbar syndrome as 'symptoms that originate in the lumbosacral region, but may extend as far as the foot'. This classification has no value because, as Mooney (1983) states, the two main reasons for a classification are first to establish a prognosis and second to provide a rationale for therapy.

5.3 The three syndromes

5.3.1 *The postural syndrome*
This is caused by mechanical deformation of soft tissues as a result of postural stresses. Prolonged maintenance of particular postures or positions which place some soft tissues under stress, will eventually produce pain. The pain ceases only with a change of position or after postural correction, thus the pain is intermittent.

The Characteristics of the postural syndrome are:

(1)   patient is usually less than 30 years of age;

(2)   usually has a sedentary occupation or lacks exercise;

(3)   pain is frequently felt in more than one area of the spine;

(4)   patients often have periods without pain;

(5)   pain relieved by change in position/posture;

(6)   pain is produced by positions not movements;

(7)   pain is intermittent;

(8)   there is no loss of movement, the patient is often hypermobile;

(9)   pain is never referred;

(10)   no signs and no pathology.

Postual neglect has two consequences. Initially there is pain without loss of function. This leads to adaptive shortening and dysfunction.

5.3.2 *The dysfunction syndrome*

This develops as a result of poor postural habit, arthropathy, trauma or derangement. The dysfunction syndrome is the condition in which adaptive shortening and resultant loss of mobility causes pain before achievement of normal end range movement. Essentially, the condition arises because movement is performed inadequately during periods of soft tissue contraction, i.e. during the healing process or during periods of immobility.

McKenzie identifies two categories of dysfunction. First, the patient who has suffered a derangement or direct trauma to the back. In this case the patient is aware of the cause of the ensuing dysfunction. He will describe the original incident as the cause. However, the original trauma or derangement will no longer be present and the symptoms will now be the result of residual loss of mobility and function. The second category is the patient who has the dysfunction as a result of poor posture or an arthrosis/arthritis. In this case the patient will be unaware of the onset. He will be unable to relate the cause of the pain to a specific incident.

The characteristics of the dysfunction syndrome are:

(1) age usually greater than 30 years old except where trauma is the predominant causitive agent;

(2) slow onset for no apparent reason;

(3) always reduced movement or function;

(4) deformity is not a principle feature, except in the elderly;

(5) test movements reproduce pain;

(6) pain is not worsened as a result of test movements;

(7) pain is felt at or just before the end of the available range of movement;

(8) as time passes morning stiffness lasts longer;

(9) the patient feels better on the move than at rest;

(10) pain is intermittent and local, occurring only when shortened tissues are placed under stress;

(11) pain sometimes comes in an episodic manner, mimicking derangement (this episodic pain is triggered by excessive use);

(12) pain is not referred except with an adherent nerve root;

(13)   a partial articular pattern is usually present if the dysfunction is due to derangement or trauma;

(14)   a full articular pattern will usually be present if the dysfunction is due to an arthrosis or arthritis.

5.3.3 *The derangement syndrome*

McKenzie defines a derangement as: 'The situation in which the normal resting position of the articular surfaces of two adjacent vertebrae is disturbed as a result of a change in position of the fluid-filled nucleus between the surfaces. The alteration of position may disturb the annular material. This change within the joint will affect the ability of the joint surfaces to move in their normal relative pathways and departures from these pathways are frequently seen. In some patients movements may only be reduced but in others they will be lost entirely' (McKenzie, 1981).

The characteristics of the derangement syndrome are:

(1)   age commonly between 20 and 55 years old;

(2)   invariably poor sitting posture;

(3)   pain of sudden onset;

(4)   pain may take 2 or 3 days to reach its peak;

(5)   often occurs for no apparent reason;

(6)   pain felt locally may radiate distally;

(7)   pain, paraestheias, or numbness may be experienced;

(8)   symptoms are directly influenced by movement;

(9)   pain may alter in respect of pain intensity or extent of pain distribution;

(10)   pain may cross the mid-line;

(11)   pain is frequently constant;

(12)   there may be no position of complete relief;

(13)   pain is usually described as an ache;

(14)   kyphosis/scoliosis deformities occur frequently;

(15)   there will usually be loss of movement or function.

5.4 **Repeated movements**

Assessment of repeated movements cannot begin before base levels of the patient's signs and symptoms in the standing position and, later on, whilst

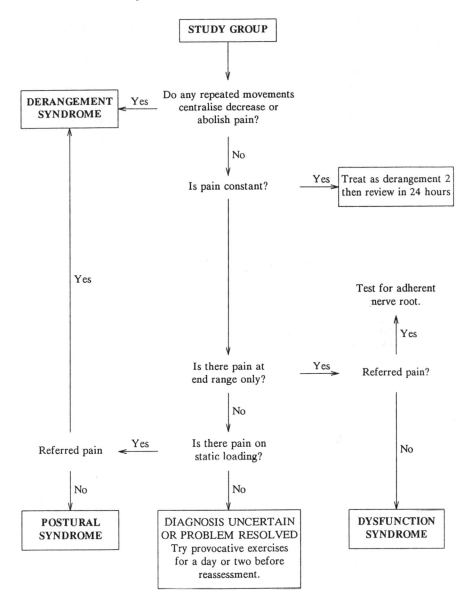

Fig. 5.1 The McKenzie assessment flow chart

lying, are accurately established. The therapist is particularly interested in the behaviour of range of movement, pain intensity, and pain distribution. In order that the therapist can describe precisely what is happening during examination, specific terms are used to describe pain behaviour (see

Appendix). McKenzie (1981) gives a detailed description of the standard repeated movements.

Interpretation of repeated movements is not easy. If it were just a case of finding out whether or not pain was felt at the end of movement, or during movement, and the effect of repetition of the movement on the pain, we would have no problem. Unfortunately, this is not the case.

In order to model the interpretation of repeated movements, and also to allow inter-therapist evaluation for research purposes, a flow chart was developed so that, by following the chart, the logic behind the assessment of repeated movements will become apparent. Figure 5.1 shows the decision-making process up to the level of the syndromes. Figure 5.2 shows the decision-making process involved in arriving at the subdivisions of the derangement syndrome.

An analogy may be drawn with organic chemistry; when extracting fractions of a complicated mixture of chemicals, the most volatile components come off first. In our case the most volatile response to repeated movements are those of patients suffering from the derangement syndrome, where it is rarely difficult either to produce or to increase pain

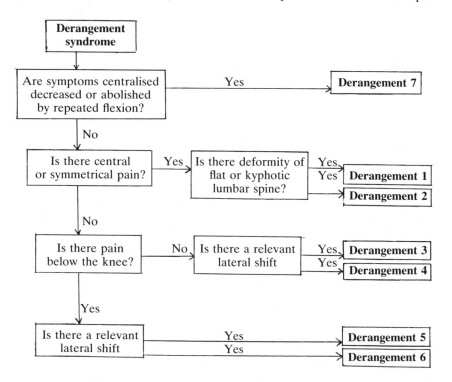

Fig. 5.2 The McKenzie derangement flow chart

in response to repeated movements. Alternatively, it is also often easy to decrease, abolish or centralise pain in response to repeated movement in a direction that reduces the derangement. Hence at the start of our flow chart, we attempt to extract as many derangements as possible by asking the question: 'Do any repeated movements decrease, abolish, or centralise pain?' If the answer is 'yes' then the patient enters the derangement flow chart (Figure 5.2) directly.

Having highlighted all easily identifiable derangements any factor that does not fit into the other two syndromes must now be extracted. Neither dysfunction nor postural syndromes cause patients to suffer constant pain. Hence the next question is: 'Is the pain constant?'

What sort of problem may lead to constant pain? Constant pain may be suffered by an individual whose annular wall has been breached. There may be sequestrated disc material, a block to extension and constant limb pain (Kopp *et al.*, 1986). The patient will probably be unable to find relief either by position or movement. A second type of problem that may end up down this arm of the flow chart is simple acute mechanical central or bilateral back ache (lumbago). Here, although all movements may increase or worsen pain, sustained positioning slowly working towards extension, may cause centralisation, or decrease, or even abolition of the pain. Such a patient usually has either a flat or kyphotic lumbar spine and would, once identified, fall into the category of derangement 2. The third type of patient who may fall into this category are those suffering from an active inflammatory disease or serious pathology. These patients should, in theory, never reach the physiotherapy department but often they do.

Entering the main trunk of the flow chart we have extracted all those cases where pain has been centralised, reduced or abolished as a result of repeated movement, as well as those with constant pain. The next task is to try to extract all cases of dysfunction. The main characteristic of dysfunctional problems, as far as repeated movements are concerned, is that they tend to suffer pain only at the end of the available range of movement. The increased pain at end range movement is not normally worsened by repetition. Derangements also may suffer end range pain on movement. However, they should have been extracted from the flow chart already.

Some cases of end range pain will have referred pain. Once again, by definition, these cannot be cases of the dysfunction syndrome. All cases with referred pain occurring at end range only should then be tested for adherent nerve root. It is at this level that the patient's history and observation of posture and movement can be helpful. An adherent nerve root is unlikely to occur in a patient suffering his first bout of pain who has a very short history of back problems. McKenzie also states that all cases of nerve root entrapment show deviation to the side of pain. The response of the patient to flexion in standing and flexion in lying helps identify an adherent nerve root. It is hypothesised by McKenzie that if pain is experienced in both the above conditions then the problem must be a disc bulging. On the other hand, if only flexion in standing is painful then the problem may be an adherent nerve root. The hypothesis works well in clinical practice.

All cases of only end range pain, without referred pain, reaching this level in the flow chart are considered to be dysfunctional problems.

If the patient does not have pain only at end range, the problem that the patient has is increasingly hard to identify. In an attempt to extract all cases of postural problems the question is asked: 'Is there pain on static loading?' If there is not, then it must be concluded that the diagnosis is uncertain or the problem has resolved. In these cases provocative exercises for 2–3 days may bring to light the cause of the pain. With some postural problems that are difficult to provoke the diagnosis may have to be made using the history. For example, the problem may only arise if the patient sits in a particular chair for three hours, before the onset of pain.

If there is pain on static loading then, by definition, the problem can only be postural, assuming there is no referred pain. If referred pain is produced on static loading, then the the problem must have been a derangement after all.

All three syndromes, or diagnostic categories, have now been extracted, as well as all cases that do not conform to the flow chart. The second flow chart is concerned with the subdivisions of the derangement syndrome.

5.5 Subdivisions of the derangement syndrome

First the unusual derangement must be dealt with, that is derangement 7, the anterior derangement. This is the only derangement where repeated flexion causes centralisation, decrease or abolition of pain.

If there is no centralisation, decrease or abolition of pain on flexion, then the derangement must be somewhere between 1 and 6, which are all posterior or posterolateral derangements. Derangements 1 to 6 are classified according to the distribution of pain, and the presence or absence of relevant spinal deformity. Derangements 1 and 2 both have central or symmetrical pain. The factor differentiating derangement 2 from 1 is that derangement 2 has the deformity of flat or kyphotic lumbar spine, and a concomitant restriction of extension of the lumbar spine.

Derangements 3 to 6 all have unilateral or assymetrical pain. Derangements 3 and 4 have pain that does not extend below the knee. The differentiating factor between derangements 3 and 4 is that derangement 4 has a relevant lateral shift and derangement 3 does not.

Derangements 5 and 6 both have pain extending below the knee.

However, derangement 6 has a relevant lateral shift and derangement 5 does not.

Work by Kilby *et al.* (1988) identified presence or absence of a relevant lateral shift as the most unreliable part of classification of the subdivisions of derangement. The presence of a visual shift or deviation to one side does not necessarily mean that a lateral component will be required to reduce the derangement. On the other hand there may be situations where a visible shift is not apparent where a lateral component is necessary to reduce the derangement. This problem is still being investigated. McKenzie considers a lateral shift to be relevant 'when the movement of side gliding alters the site of intensity of the pain'. In practice the situation is not so clear cut.

Having identified the diagnostic categories and subdivisions, what relevance do they have to prognosis and rationale for therapy?

5.6 Rationale for therapy

5.6.1 *Postural syndrome*
A patient with postural syndrome will recover if taught how to avoid placing prolonged stresses on the structures causing their postural pain. The process of postural re-education can have almost immediate effects. The difficult part of the treatment is often motivating the patient enough to persist with their own treatment. It is the patient who is solving their own problem by self-treatment, the therapist only supplies the explanation of the problem and the means of recovery. The patient must take responsibility for their own problem. Although postural pain can be relieved fairly rapidly, it may take several weeks for the sensitivity of the overstressed structures to fall to a normal level. Therefore, exacerbation of the pain initially occurs readily when the patient lapses into their old habits. Given time, and continual self-correction, sensitivity to pain is lost and new postural habits learnt.

5.6.2 *Dysfunction syndrome*
The principle of treatment for the dysfunctional problem is to stretch contracted soft tissues in a controlled manner so enabling the patient once again to achieve a full painless range of movement in all directions without micro-trauma. Once again the patient is given an explanation of the problem and how it has probably come about. They are then taught how to begin to solve the problem for themselves. The patient is started on self-treatment, and only if this is not proving sucessful is a therapist technique used. Treatment may take 4–6 weeks to achieve its objective. However, once the patient has been seen a few times and the therapist is sure he or she is safe, is improving, and knows what to look for if things are going

wrong, he may be left for considerable periods to work on his own. The therapist is always available at the end of the phone. Patients are always warned that they will experience new pains during and after exercise. If no pain is produced during performance of exercise for the recovery of lost movement, the contracted tissues are not being stretched enough to enhance elongation of shortened structures. On the other hand if pain persists at an elevated level for more than 10 to 20 min on completion of exercise, the exercise has been too vigorous.

5.6.3 *Derangement syndrome*

The principle of treatment for derangement is to encourage the patient to reduce their own derangement by the use of exercises tailored to their particular derangement. Once reduction of derangement has been achieved, the patient must be taught how to maintain the reduction. Once the reduction is stable, recovery of function can be worked on. From the onset treatment runs side by side with an explanation of the cause and also of the treatment methods. Self-treatment is attempted before any pure therapist technique is used. Self-reliance must be inculcated in order that recurrence is prevented. Exercises for derangement are, as a general rule, performed in the direction that causes centralisation, decrease or abolition of pain. This is diametrically opposed to the treatment of dysfunction which is aimed at the painful restricted movements. It can be seen therefore that if the diagnosis is wrong the treatment will either be ineffective or make the problem worse. This problem is tackled in two ways. First, patients are always briefed on what they should experience and also what they may feel if the problem should worsen or the 'pain pattern' extends. They are then told the appropriate action to take.

5.7 **Prognostic value of examination findings**

At present I am not aware of any research into the prognostic value of examination findings or duration of problem in the postural or dysfunction syndromes. As a general rule with the derangement syndrome, the further into the lower limb the referred pain extends, the slower the reduction or poorer the expected outcome of treatment. Most physiotherapy findings are purely empirical. There is one paper by Kopp *et al.* (1986) that highlights the importance of lumbar extension as a predictor of outcome. Their research was retrospective and, as such, would not be expected to be as accurate as a prospective study. Of the 67 patients who met the criteria for inclusion in the study, 35 patients were treated without operation, of these, 97% were able to achieve normal lumbar extension within 3 days of admission to hospital. Unfortunately Kopp did not comment on any concomitant centralisation of pain. In his study, 32 patients underwent laminectomy and discectomy because they failed to improve with conservative measures. Of the 32 patients requiring surgery, only two were able to achieve normal lumbar extension preoperatively (it would be interesting to know if these two patients showed centralisation or not). The authors recommended the use of extension exercises. The paper goes on to discuss the relative merits of McKenzie's and Williams' exercises in the treatment of low back pain, relating the theory of disc migration with movement, the pathology, and the intradiscal pressures in various positions.

The other predictor of good results with derangements is the centralisation phenomenon. Donelson *et al.* (1986) state that: 'the occurrence of centralisation is absolutely reliable in determining appropriate treatment and predicting outcome'. Donelson's study was retrospective. They found that, out of a sample size of 87 patients, 59 had an excellent result following McKenzie treatment (excellent means complete relief from symptoms with full function) and all of these experienced centralisation of their pain. The percentage of patients showing centralisation progressively fell as the result of treatment became worse. Only 37.5% of patients with a poor result showed centralisation of pain. There is one proviso to Donelson's statement that centralisation is a good predictor of outcome. Some patients centralise in extension but cannot maintain centralisation once they move from the extended position. Failure to maintain centralisation in the first few minutes following treatment is a good predictor of failure to recover. Donelson also states that absence of centralisation is frequently an early predictor of the need for surgical treatment. This fits in with Kopp's findings because recovery of extension and centralisation frequently occur simultaneously.

5.8 Conclusions

McKenzie's three mechanical back pain syndromes, plus the rules of behaviour of the syndromes, build up into an extremely powerful model of the behaviour of back pain, especially when factors such as intradiscal pressure variations in various postures (Nachemson, 1976), together with the theory of migration of nuclear disc material (McKenzie, 1981), with maintenance of static postures are linked together.

McKenzie's treatment methods are based on the syndrome, to which patient's symptoms belong, and also on the individual patient's specific problem. It can easily be understood why a bland non-specific form of treatment, such as back school, has such a poor treatment result (Dimaggio & Mooney, 1987). If patients are to be given advice and exercises they must be tailored to the patient's individual problem.

To end on a controversial note; if the ability to extend the lumbar spine after 3 days of McKenzie treatment can, without doubt, be used as a predictor of the likely need for surgery, the amount of time physiotherapists spend treating hopeless conservative cases on the instruction of consultants could be cut dramatically. This may make the physiotherapy department very unpopular with the referring medical practitioners. However, it may force radical changes in the way the majority of orthopaedic surgeons manage their problem back pain patients. Surely if patients requiring surgery can be identified, and operated on quickly, postoperative complications will be lessened. A prospective research project aimed at determining the reliability of inability to extend and or lack of centralisation of pain, following McKenzie treatment, as a predictor of the need for surgical intervention could have tremendous implications.

References

Dimaggio, A. & Mooney, V. (1987a), Conservative care for low back pain: what works? *The Journal of Musculoskeletal Medicine*, **4**, 27–34.

Dimaggio, A. & Mooney, V. (1987b), The McKenzie program: exercise effective against back pain, *The Journal of Musculoskeletal Medicine*, **4**, 63–74.

Donelson, R., Silva, G. & Murphy, K. (1990), Centralization phenomenon. Its usefulness in evaluating and treating referred pain, *Spine*, **15**, 211–13.

Kopp, J. R., Alexander, A.H., Turosy, R.H., Leverini, M.G. & Lichtman, D.M. (1986), The use of lumbar extension in the evaluation and treatment of patients with acute herniated nucleus pulposus: a preliminary report, *Clinical Orthopaedics and Related Research*, **202**, 211–8.

Mc Kenzie, R. A. (1981), *The Lumbar Spine Mechanical Diagnosis and Therapy*, Spinal Publications Limited, Wellington, New Zealand.

Mooney, V. (1983), The syndromes of low back disease. In: *The Orthopaedic Clinics of North America*, Guest Editor V. Mooney, **14**, 505–15. W.B. Saunders Company, Philadelphia.

Nachemson, A.L. (1976), The lumbar spine, an orthopaedic challenge, *Spine*, **1**, 59.

Nwuga, G. & Nwuga, V. (1985), Relative therapeutic efficacy of the Williams and McKenzie protocols in back pain management, *Physiotherapy Practice*, 99–105.

Ponte, D. J., Jensen, G. J., & Kent, B. E. (1984), A preliminary report on the use of the McKenzie protocol *versus* Williams protocol in the treatment of low back pain, *The Journal of Orthopaedic and Sports Physical Therapy*, **6**, 130–8.

Appendix. Terms used to describe pain behaviour with movement

Increase: symptoms already present are increased in intensity.

Decrease: symptoms already present are decreased in intensity.

Produced: there are no symptoms at rest. Movement creates symptoms.

Abolishes: there are symptoms at rest. Movement eliminates symptoms.

Worsens: symptoms present or produced are increased with movement and remain worse as a result.

Not worsened: symptoms present or produced are increased with each movement, but do not remain worse as a result.

Better: symptoms present or produced are decreased or abolished with movement, and remain better as a result.

No better: symptoms that are decreased or abolished with movement do not remain decreased or abolished.

Pain during movement: pain appears or increases as movement occurs. Pain disappears or reduces when movement stops.

Pain at end range: pain does not appear until end range is reached. Pain disappears or reduces on return to neutral position.

In status quo: movement has no effect on the patient's symptoms.

Centralisation: movement of referred pain from a distal to a more proximal part of the limb, buttock or back, in the case of the lumbar spine.

Peripheralisation: movement of pain from a proximal to a more distal part of the limb.

Full Articular Pattern or Capsular Pattern (cyriax term): of limitation of movement is a set proportion of limited passive movements in a joint, invariable for one particular joint, but different from one joint to another. In the case of the spine there is equal limitation in all directions. The finding of a capsular pattern on examination indicates that the lesion present is an arthritis or osteoarthrosis of the joint.

Partial Articular Pattern or Non-Capsular Pattern (Cyriax term): This occurs when limitation of movement at a particular joint is found not to conform with the known capsular pattern. The origin can be:

　internal derangement
　ligamentous or capsular adhesions
　extra-articular.

Discussion

Fairbank: This is quite a different approach, from those we have heard today, to the analysis of what I think is a specific section of the back pain population. How do you see the patients that you are talking about relating to those that previous speakers have been describing?

Stigant (in reply): The patients that can be treated using the McKenzie techniques are in general not those patients that the surgeon would consider operating on for prolapsed intervertebral disc, spinal stenosis or bony instability. The patients responding to McKenzie type treatment have one factor in common, one or more of the standard repeated movements will cause centralisation, decrease or abolition of pain in the case of the derangement syndrome; an increase of pain at end of the available range of movement in the case of the dysfunction syndrome. There are no signs and no symptoms on examination in the case of the postural syndrome.

Fairbank: So you are really saying that this classification is based on 'response to treatment'?

Stigant (in reply): Yes, in so much that the repeated movements used to initially assess the patient are also the movements that are used to treat the patient. During the assessment the therapist is looking for movements that will cause a beneficial change in the patient signs and symptoms. It may happen that during the course of the initial assessment the patient may be rendered pain free due to the assessment procedure in mild cases of the derangement syndrome.

Fairbank: Is it possible then, if looking at the response to treatment, to see how reliable these three main groups are? If the only way you can identify which group a patient falls into is by treating the patient, then presumably you cannot get another observer to come along and then say whether they would have put them in the same group.

Stigant (in reply): We have actually looked at the inter-therapist reliability when using the McKenzie assessment of patients, using the assessment flow chart described. Using two therapists, one to directly assess the patient and the other observing and noting the patient's responses to questioning. It was possible post assessment for the therapists to be assessed blindly by an adjudicator on their responses to the questions on the flow chart, thus allowing inter-therapist reliability to be established.

Fairbank: Are you able to give us numbers?

Stigant (in reply): They were presented at the November 1988 meeting of the Society for Back Pain Research as a poster (Kilby J., Stigant M. and Roberts A., Assessing Physical Therapy Assessments: A McKenzie Algorithm). (This is shown on Table 5.1.)

Mitchell: Having listened for most of the morning to increasingly complex mathematical data and classification of syndromes, it seems that the McKenzie classification is steeped in the mystery of physiotherapy rather than numbers. The

Table 5.1   Reliability study of McKenzie assessments

Element of flow chart	Number of pairs of observations	Percentage agreement
Do any repeated movements decrease, centralise or abolish the pain?	41	90
Is the pain constant?	1	95
Pain at end range only?	0	70
Referred pain?	4	100
Pain on static loading?	9	100
Are symptoms centralised, decreased or abolished by repeated flexion?	16	100
Central/symmetrical pain?	15	93.3
Pain below the knee?	9	100
Deformity of flat or kyphotic lumbar spine?	5	80
Relevant lateral shift?	9	55

use of the words 'may', 'maybe', 'frequently' and 'not frequently' are apparent. Basically, how reliable are the various physiotherapists who classify the patients. You use the words 'fairly reliable', and it seems as if numbers would make it a lot more easy for us to understand.

Stigant (in reply): I would love to put numbers to the reliability of various physiotherapists classifying patients. However, at the moment physiotherapy research in this area is embryonic. As researchers we have established one method of looking at inter-therapist reliability. Extending this process to look at the reliability of physiotherapists during normal departmental work would prove very interesting. Given time, general figures for assessment reliability will be available.

Swannell: I just wonder if you could tell us how many patients, roughly, fall outside this classification system?

Stigant (in reply): It depends on the sort of population of patients you have got. Of the patients actually coming into the department where I work, I would say that maybe 70% fall within this category.

Fairbank: Where do these patients come from?

Stigant (in reply): Mainly orthopaedic surgeons, with a few General Practice referrals.

Fairbank: Everybody is talking about different groups of patients seen from their own particular angle. Dr Barker has already made it very clear that he is looking at a different population from that which I am seeing as an orthopaedic surgeon.

John: McKenzie started his programme of investigation of his methods in 1963, and first published papers in 1968. He has trained many thousands of physiotherapists and doctors. Nachemson has produced evidence of the efficacy of the extension and centralisation method of diagnosis. It is a method which does allow the specification of non-mechanical back pain symptoms, once the medical profession has excluded other pathological conditions.

McKenzie R. A. (1972), Manual correction of sciatic scoliosis, *The New Zealand Medical Journal*, **76**, 194–9.
McKenzie R. A. (1979), Prophylaxis in recurrent low back pain, *New Zealand Medical Journal*, **89**.

Nelson (to Mrs John): In your opinion, how good is the medical profession in selecting patients for your clearly very successful treatment? We would like to try and establish what number of patients fall into the category that you can treat. You have given us a little clue, but I would question how good doctors are at selection, and I would suggest that you are still receiving a very broad mixed hotch-potch of all sorts.

John (in reply): I would accept, Mr Nelson, your comment but I think we can positively say that through the McKenzie examination and with the co-operation of our medical colleagues, we can hope to exclude patients whom we suspect of having pathological conditions. There is a large percentage of mechanical low back pain which can be treated and is directed to us from general practitioners and other orthopaedic surgeons as well as through self-referral.

Humphrey: In this classificaiton, is there any attempt to identify the lesion or site of lesion?

Stigant (in reply): We cannot say for sure exactly where the lesion is.

An osteopathic view of back pain classification

6.1 Introduction

This chapter will be not so much an osteopathic classification of back pain as a general appraisal of the subject from a viewpoint that takes account of osteopathic concepts and experience.

For practical purposes, a system of classification is a tool to analyse variability and make predictions. The value of any tool lies solely in its ability to perform its allotted task which, in classifications of disease, is primarily the prediction of outcome and response to treatment. The requisite tool will, therefore, vary somewhat according to the therapeutic range of the practitioner employing it. There has been a tendency to concentrate on the classification of individuals into diagnostic groups, which is useful if groups can be easily recognised that have marked differences in prognosis and response to the therapies available. This chapter will seek to show that such a classification is not invariably appropriate, and that it may be an obstacle to progress in the research and treatment of back pain.

6.2 Background

Historically the most effective classification into diagnostic groups has been that made according to pathological process and its anatomical site; by identifying these two features it was often found that a disease could be defined and its natural history and response to treatment predicted. Following this principle a taxonomical juggernaut, directed mainly by morbid anatomists following Virchow, has rolled on for a century or more and produced an impressive disease catalogue. In situations where a condition has defied the histologists, distinct patterns of clinical features have been used to identify a disease entity, usually in the belief that these syndromes have an underlying morbid anatomical basis awaiting demonstration.

It seems that this classification system has achieved such status in medical thinking that for many the obvious approach to understanding maladies affecting any region or system of the body is to list the structures involved, subdivided into the possible pathological processes which might affect each, and try to fit every clinical presentation into one of the classes so formed. There is no lack of such classifications in the literature on back pain.

6.3 **Present practice**

To some extent, osteopathy has accommodated itself to this system by using the extension of the definition of pathology favoured by Wyke. He recognises both *structural pathology*, in which morbid anatomical processes have produced tissue change observable at least histologically, and *functional pathology* in which symptoms and disability arise from dysfunctioning structures without even histological change. Both Wyke (1987) and most osteopaths (MacDonald & Peters, 1986) consider that the bulk of back pain is caused by functional pathology, and many will classify their patients by the type of dysfunction and its anatomical location.

Although most medical practitioners are uncertain whether to accept dysfunction as an independent entity, and therefore do not accept the major part of osteopathic thinking, a *modus vivendi* has arisen between much of orthodoxy and osteopathy. This depends on the two groups accepting a demarcation on opposite sides of which each can use its own classification system to select patients for its own range of treatments. In the interests of harmony, and to foster a complementary relationship, inconsistencies in this approach are not stressed by either side.

The demarcation between problems deemed to be caused by structural as opposed to functional pathology is generally arrived at from the history and standard clinical examination. Following that initial decision, conventional medicine focuses most diagnostic attention on those cases involving a structural pathology for which definitive treatments are available; both the diagnostic facilities necessary, and the treatments indicated, tend to be hospital-based and therefore irrelevant to osteopathic practice. The remainder of 'non-specific' or 'mechanical' patients have no proven remedies available within conventional medicine and are therefore not differentiated by most orthopaedic and rheumatological specialists; they are often referred *en masse* for unspecified physiotherapy.

Meanwhile, many osteopaths will refer to conventional medicine those patients whose symptoms clearly derive from a structural pathological process while focussing their discriminatory efforts on the other side of the demarcation line. The range of functional pathology will be classified by spinal level or muscle group, and by motion restriction, inappropriate position, or abnormal tissue texture or tenderness; this classification is made in terms that would convey little meaning to non-osteopaths. Much of this classification process uses pattern recognition skills which take time and training to develop, but its purpose is selection for specific manipulations so that it has little utility for those who are not going to use these treatments.

Thus, by using the agreed demarcation line and classifying patients by pathological process and its location, orthodoxy and osteopathy can be complementary to each other in what could be termed a collusive compromise involving a measure of intellectual apartheid. However, as our approach to back pain becomes more knowledgeable and sophisticated, for both disciplines this system becomes more obviously inadequate.

6.4 Critique

For conventional doctors the most obvious problem to emerge is the weak predictive value of observed structural pathology for either extent of pain or response to surgery or other treatment. While the majority of sufferers from back pain defy attempts to demonstrate a structural pathology that could cause their symptoms and disability, even when such pathology is found, we are warned against using it to define the patient's condition, by Duncan Troup's statement of 1977: 'Practically every single morbid pathological change to which back or sciatic pain has been ascribed has later been demonstrated in the symptom-free'. Therefore, because the presence of structural pathology cannot alone predict symptomatic back problems, nor the absence of such pathology predict comfort, other determinants have been sought. Identifying adverse factors in the realms of cognition, emotion, function and behaviour, has offered welcome prospects of benefit from their modification. Less welcome, however, as we learn more about how to quantify these factors is the realisation that they occur independently of the classification above; so the likelihood of its becoming an efficient predictive tool, even following the advent of more structural pathological data, becomes increasingly remote.

In the face of such difficulties, the perceived necessity to classify individual back pain sufferers into groups should be examined.

Relevant here is the common prejudice that the process of classifying any range of phenomena into groups with similar properties is the precursor to knowledge about them. The archetype of such systems, the Linneaen classification of living things, is probably the influential model. In Figure 6.1 such a classification is represented as a branched system; each significant factor excluding the possibility of some classes and raising the

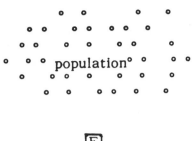

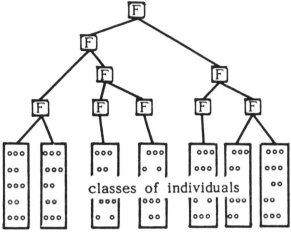

Fig. 6.1 Diagram of classification on the Linnaean model: each discriminatory factor (F) allows selection from its dependent branches and subsequent repetition of this process eventually separates the population into classes of individuals with ranges of features in common

probability of those at the end of the branch selected, until, as a terminal twig is reached, the probability of that class becomes unity and that of all other classes nil. The species genotype predicts the bulk of the features of individuals who can belong to only one such class, e.g. a whelk will always be more like other whelks than like any ant. To arrive at a diversity of such distinct classes a branched decision system seems inevitable. However, the special properties of these classes – mutually exclusive, permanent, and highly predictive – do not prevail in most other situations where classifications operate, so that for these the use of Linnaean classification as a model will always be an exercise in analogy

This analogy will seem most apt when the features of the disease are largely determined by the pathology and different structural pathologies seldom coexist in the same patient. Thus, when many diseases were incurable and severely affected individuals for the remainder of their lives, the analogy could be extended to consider sufferers almost as a sub-species of *Homo sapiens*: the consumptive, the syphilitic, the leper, etc. However, pathological processes do not put such an indelible imprint on the future history of individuals as do specific genotypes, so that, when other strong determinants of outcome exist, and different pathologies coexist, the analogy must be expected to break down, and this classification become a poor predictor. In this situation no natural law has been overturned; simply a different tool to analyse variability is needed.

6.5 A multifactorial classification

The only method of using past experience to predict outcome and treatment response in back pain may be not to classify individuals into groups, but to classify the range of determinants which may increase liability to back pain and assess their relative contribution to each sufferer's experience. From such studies, groups of individuals might subsequently be identified, but this is not essential.

In Figure 6.2 such a classification is represented diagrammatically; a range of factors is seen influencing each individual.

In Table 6.1 an attempt has been made to draft such a classification for back pain. While it is beyond the scope of this chapter to justify the

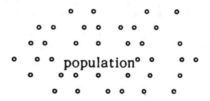

classification of factors

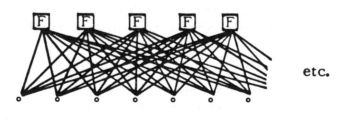

etc.

individuals

Fig. 6.2   Diagram of multifactorial classification system; for each individual, the influence of each of a range of factors with predictive power (F) is acknowledged

Table 6.1   Factors in low back pain generation

1. *Structural Anomalies*
   1.1 Leg length inequality
   1.2 Healed fracture with angulation
   1.3 Asymmetrical facets, unilateral
       sacralisation or lumbarisation
   1.4 Scheuermann disease, etc.

2. *Postural Abnormality*
   Causes   – False perception of ideal posture
            – Inadequate postural skills
            – Inadequate muscle power
            – Involuntary muscle action:
                anxiety patterns
                pain response (9.1)
                abnormal function (8.1)
            – Restriction of range of motion of joints (1.2, 1.4, 3.4, 4.4)

   Effects 2.1 Excess lordosis (a) lumbar (b) high thoracic
            2.2 Excess thoracic or thoraco-lumbar kyphosis
            2.3 Slow onset loss of range of movement

3. *Misuse*
   Causes   – Ignorance of good use
            – External constraints: social, ergonomic
            – Inappropriate response to pain:
                immobility
                stoicism

   Effects 3.1 muscle fatigue
            3.2 excessive compressive forces generated
            3.3 excessive tension generated
            3.4 immobility effects

4. *Disc*
   Causes   – excess load; acute or repetitive (3.2, 1.3)
            – immobility effects (3.4, 2.3)

   Effects 4.1 internal derangement – possible outer annular pain generation
            4.2 herniation
            4.3 prolapse
            4.4 loss of mobility

5. *Reduced Posterior Compartment Space*
   Causes   – congenital
            – reduced disc height (4.1–4.3)
            – facet osteophytes
            – spondylolisthesis
            – hyperextension of joint
                postural (2.1)
                misuse (3.2)
                muscle tension (8.1)

Table 6.1   Cont

_____

                        − space occupying body
                          e.g. neuroma

Effects   5.1 root and dural sleeve pressure
            5.2 pressure on other nerves to produce
                 either, (a) reduced A inhibitory, or
                 (b) ectopic C excitatory, impulses
            5.3 compression of other tissues
                 e.g. interspinous ligaments

6. *Nerve Roots and Dural Sleeve*
    Causes   − pressure from disc (4.2, 4.3)
              − encroachment from reduced posterior compartment dimension
              (5.1)

    Effects   6.1 pain
              6.2 paraesthesiae
              6.3 deficits

7. *Sacro-iliac Joint*
              7.1 hypermobility
              7.2 painful hypomobility
              7.3 painless hypomobility
              7.4 inflammatory arthritis

8. *Abnormal Function*
    Causes   − reflex to nociceptor afferents (9.2)
              − facilitated by abnormal afferent traffic
              − altered spinal reflexes (9.4)
              − abnormal patterns generated
              − inappropriate patterns generated
              − proprioceptor malfunction
              − 'joint bind'? meniscoids and synovial folds

    Effects   8.1 increased muscle tension: segmental (a)
                                               group   (b)
              8.2 decreased joint motion: segmental (a)
                                               group   (b)
              8.3 abnormal axes of joint motion
              8.4 abnormal forces generated

(*Note*: Myofascial pain and dysfunction, MPD, in gluteal muscles commonly a
differential diagnostic factor as pain is experienced in buttock and leg, in common
with many low back pain situations.)

9. *Nociceptor Excitation*
    Causes
    Chemical   − in abnormally active muscle (8.1, 3.1)
                 − in tissue damage: (a) trauma, (b) morbid anatomical changes
    Mechanical   − compression (2.1, 5.1, 5.3, 6.1, 8.4), gravity
                 − tension (3.3, 2.2, 8.4), abnormal muscle action

Table 6.1   Cont.

Effects	9.1 spinothalamic outflow, pain awareness
	9.2 reflex effects on muscles
	9.3 reflex effects on other organs
	9.4 altered spinal reflexes, 'spinal fixation'

10. *Modulation*

    Causes – reduced A inhibitory inflow (2.3, 3.4, 4.4, 5.2a, 8.2)

               – reduced EMAS activity

               – emotional mechanisms: anxiety

                                      depression

inclusion of each item, they are generally supported by documented clinical evidence or derive from physiological data; very few are controversial. Of more importance than the validity of each item is their relationship to each other. Hardly any are mutually exclusive. Very few are strong enough predictors for back pain that they are likely to be its sole cause. While each has at least some independence of the others, interaction is inevitable with summation, synergistic and positive feed-back effects all possible. The classification allows for an infinitely variable multi-factorial aetiology, with most factors indicating specific treatments which may be put together in a multifaceted prescription. There may be individuals in whom very few adverse factors determine most of the characteristics of their disease, e.g. an acute large disc herniation compressing a dural sleeve in an individual of previously robust physical and mental health. Such patients might be successfully managed by assessing and treating one factor only, but these should not be considered the 'typical' cases of homogeneous groups to be defined ever more accurately by data: they are more likely to be atypical in their paucifactorial pathogenesis.

The proposed system's flexibility is such that the possibility of other more rigid systems occurring within it is not excluded. The onus is therefore on those who propose more constrained systems to prove their efficiency in accounting for variability. Justification of this alternative classification by data is difficult, due to its complexity, but Kuhn proposes that, in adopting a different conceptual model, established observations and experiments change their significance (Kuhn, 1970). The test of the conceptual model is whether it provides better explanations for these observations than models used hitherto.

6.6 Application of proposed classification system

To illustrate this we might look critically at the DHSS Working Group on Back Pain report of 1979, which says: 'Back pain ... is therefore heterogeneous. Failure to delineate distinct syndromes retards both the search for aetiological insights and the evaluation of different approaches to treatment', and, 'Although crude classifications have been employed, these have proved to be insufficiently precise to produce satisfactory homogeneous sub-groups for trials.' Thus variability of outcome is seen by many researchers to be due to the admixture of a variety of classes of back pain each with a different natural history, and they continue to search for the criteria to recognise these classes. However, by applying the alternative model, we can question the presumption that 'distinct syndromes' and 'homogeneous sub-groups' exist. Acceptance of the possibility that they may not exist, would lead to trial designs in which more effort was made to quantify, or to eliminate or otherwise control for, the several factors in each case which may be determining outcome other than the test variable. It is noteworthy that none of the reports of trials of manipulation for back pain over the last 20 years specify the instructions given to patients concerning physical activity and pain response strategies.

The present approach to selection for surgery for back problems can be discussed in terms of the multifactorial classification of patients. Apart from the impending loss of bladder innervation by cauda equina compression, there is probably no absolute structural pathological surgical indication. As surgical practice evolves, although new imaging techniques are dramatically enhancing the precision of anatomical assessment, improvement in operative success rates is being achieved more by considering other features of the patient's situation. Practising surgeons, even when relying on ill-defined personal judgement, often take account of disability indices, psychological inventories, and especially the response to activity restriction. The latter measure is a means of cancelling the effects of many factors related to body-use, occupation, muscle spasm, and some aspects of mental stress, and thereby attempts to reveal the contribution of structural pathology to the patient's pain and disability. The usefulness of this process is such that few surgeons would think it worthwhile to seek anatomical information beyond the scope of plain radiology, until some trial of rest had taken place.

I think that we can argue from logic and present data for our classification of significant factors rather than of individuals, but the relationships of the various factors, the systems into which they may be linked, offer many possibilities for hypotheses and experimental investigation. It is an inclusive model so that all the present rival theories can be proposed within its terms of reference. In its multifactorial approach and necessity of assessing each sufferer individually, it coincidentally will appeal to those espousing holistic principles.

For osteopaths the classification is fertile conjectural ground. They see day-to-day variation in pain and disability shadowing the variations in the tactile and visual signs of dysfunction that they assess. The rapid fluctuations observed seem to follow physical activity and perhaps emotion; slower trends follow structural pathologies, habitual body-use, anatomical variations, etc. (MacDonald, 1988). A hypothetical system which accords with this experience, is of pain production within dysfunctioning muscles or structures on which their excessive tensions act, with the muscle dysfunction persisting partly by a reflex pain/spasm/pain cycle (Roland, 1986), and also interacting with the activity of the patient according to the mathematical model previously presented to a Society for Back Pain Research meeting (MacDonald, 1985; see Appendix). Most other factors in the classification could be represented as increasing the gain or threshold of the positive feedback loops postulated.

6.7 Conclusion

An alternative classification system for back pain is proposed to allow predictions about an individual sufferer to be based on the contributions of several factors. This is deemed a more valid and useful analytical tool than one which attempts to allot individuals to diagnostic groups.

References

Department of Health and Social Security (1979), *Working Group on Back Pain*, pp. 19, 38, HMSO, London.

Kuhn, T. S. (1970), *The Structure of Scientific Revolutions*, Chicago University Press.

MacDonald, R. S. (1988), Osteopathic diagnosis of back pain, *Manual Medicine*, **3**, 110–13.

MacDonald, R. S. & Peters, D. (1986), Osteopathy, *Practitioner*, **230**, 1073–6.

Roland, M. O. (1986), A critical review of the evidence for a pain/spasm/pain cycle in spinal disorders, *Clinical Biomechanics*, **1**, 102–9.

Roland, M. O. & Morris, R. (1983), A study of the natural history of back pain. Part 1: Development of a reliable and sensitive measure of disability in low-back pain, *Spine*, **8**, 141–4.

Wiesel, S. W., Cuckler, J. M., Deluca, F., Zeide, M. S., & Rothman, R. H. (1980), Acute low-back pain. An objective analysis of conservative therapy, *Spine*, **5**, 324–30.

Wyke, B. (1987). The neurology of low back pain. In: *The Lumbar Spine and Back Pain*, ed. M. I. V. Jayson, pp 56–99, Pitman, London.

Appendix

A hypothetical mathematical model for the natural history of non-specific low back pain was presented by the author to the Society for Back Pain Research in 1985.

The severity of the back problem is represented by a variable, the Comfortable Repertoire (CR), on a continuum from 'no comfortable activities' to 'all normal activities comfortable'. [The real equivalent of CR exists as the scores of disability questionnaires such as that of Roland & Morris (1983).] A graph of the evolution of a back pain episode would show CR plotted on a vertical axis of increasing stressfulness of activities against a horizontal time axis. The actual activities performed (PA) by the patient could also be plotted on the same vertical axis. In the proposed model of back pain natural history, the rate of change in CR with respect to time is assumed to vary as the excess of CR over PA. Thus the more activities performed are within the range which is comfortable, the faster that range increases: conversely, the more stressful the activities performed outside the comfortable repertoire, the faster that repertoire diminishes. Using published data for varied rates of recovery depending on varying levels of rest (Wiesel *et al.*, 1970), and simulating realistic patient behaviour, the model predicts variation in outcome of back pain episodes at least as great as that observed clinically.

Discussion

Kirwan: Can you measure the information from the tactile sensations that you acquired?

MacDonald (in reply): If several observers make some sort of quantification, and work together for long enough, then inter-observer assessments can be reliable. It is not done very frequently.

Kirwan: It is just that your hypothesis cannot be tested unless you can measure it.

7 *K. Humphreys*

Back pain syndromes – a chiropractic perspective

7.1 Introduction

The purpose of this chapter is to present an introduction to the classification of back pain syndromes as currently taught at the Anglo-European College of Chiropractic. Although this classification system is not fully accepted by the chiropractic profession worldwide, it is representative of the direction in which chiropractic education is heading in the United Kingdom and Europe. Perhaps a useful insight into this classification system would be to state from the outset that the syndromes are categorised according to history, pain distribution, physical examination and radiographic findings. This approach intends to try to identify both the major pain source as well as the level and extent of spinal dysfunction. Therefore, this classification system is clinical in nature and is not necessarily a reflection of the true pathogenesis (Kirkaldy-Willis & Cassidy, 1985). No attempt will be made to expand upon the generally accepted concepts of inter-vertebral disc disease, spinal stenosis, instability, repetitive stress/strain injuries or spondylolisthesis. Instead, this chapter will highlight the lesser known and perhaps more controversial referred pain syndromes of spinal dysfunction, posterior facet, sacro-iliac and combined posterior facet and sacro-iliac syndromes, as well as myofascial pain syndromes. (See Table 7.1).

7.2 Dysfunction of spinal motion

Research into the functioning of the lumbar spine during coronal plane motion has revealed an association of lateral flexion and axial rotation at each vertebral level called coupled motion (Lovett, 1905; Arkin, 1950; Miles & Sullivan, 1961; Gregersen & Lucas, 1967; Frymoyer *et al.*, 1979;

Table 7.1   Classification of common back-pain syndromes

Dysfunction of spinal motion (Categories I-IV)
Posterior facet syndrome
Sacro-iliac syndrome
Combined posterior facet and sacroiliac syndromes
Myofascial pain syndromes
Intervertebral disc disease
Repetitive stress/strain injuries
Segmental instability
Lateral nerve root entrapment (recurrent dynamic, fixed)
Central spinal stenosis
Degenerative spondylolisthesis (stable, unstable)
Isthmic spondylolisthesis

Pearcy & Tibrewal, 1984). Cassidy (1976) and Grice (1979) have proposed a system containing four categories of lumbar spinal motion as detected on lateral stress X-rays. Type I is considered to be the normal coupled motion in lateral bending whereby the vertebra tilts towards the side of bending, the intervertebral disc wedges with the apex towards the bending or concave side and the vertebral body axially rotates towards the convex side. On X-ray the axial rotation is seen simply as a spinous process rotating towards the concavity. Types II-IV are categorised as aberrant movement patterns due to their variation from Type I. Type II is defined as a lack or complete reversal of the normal axial rotation associated with the lateral tilt. On X-ray this may be seen as a lack of spinous process rotation or a spinous process rotating towards the convexity of the curve. Normal disc wedging prevails in Type II. Type III is typified by normal axial rotation but the disc either fails to close or reverses so that the wedging occurs with the apex to the convexity of the curve. Type IV combines both abnormal disc wedging and abnormal axial rotation. It is essentially Type II and Type III combined. On lateral stress X-rays this is characterised by a spinous process rotation towards the con-vexity and lack of discal wedging.

Although there is no definite evidence concerning the possible progression from Type I to Type IV, it is considered that Type IV is the most serious clinical condition in this particular classification system and is commonly seen in the presence of discal pathology (Weitz, 1981). It is also thought that these aberrant motions contribute to the production of the facet syndrome (Ghormley, 1933) and degenerative disc disease, as well as being the earliest detectable changes seen on X-ray leading to the process of lumbar spondylosis (Gitelman, 1980).

The clinical picture is varied and not well defined. However, the diagnosis of spinal dysfunction is based mainly on the X-ray findings correlated with passive motion (movement palpation) tests, restriction and/or painful active lumbar movements, localised tenderness around the involved spinal levels and the absence of any neurological signs (Dupuis *et al.*, 1985). Treatment is instituted as early as possible in an attempt to restore Type I motion.

7.3 The posterior facet syndrome

It has been known for many years that the posterior facet joints of the lumbar spine are capable of producing various low back and/or leg complaints (Goldthwait, 1911; Ghormley, 1933; Badgley, 1941; Hirsch *et al.*, 1963). Since Ghormley's introduction of the term facet syndrome in 1933, general interest in the subject has waxed and waned. More recently a revived enthusiasm has produced further evidence for this clinic entity (Shealy, 1974; King & Lagger, 1976; McCall *et al.*, 1979; Fairbank *et al.*, 1981; Selby & Paris, 1981; Lippit, 1984).

The clinical features of the posterior facet syndrome are variable. This is pro-bably due to the inclusion of several distinct lesions of the facets and associated structures under the umbrella term of facet syndrome. The usual presenting complaints are of low back pain and/or referred pain into the lower extremity. The pain is an ill-defined (sclerotomal) type that may mimic radicular pain by its distribution into the buttock, posterior thigh and occasionally below the knee (Kirkaldy-Willis & Hill, 1979). Lumbar extension movements may be restricted and painful as well as combined extension and lateral rotation towards the painful side. Commonly seen is a localised tenderness and muscle spasm over the involved facet joint(s) (Gitelman, 1980). Motion palpation tests and stress lateral bending X-rays may reveal abnormal coupling motions typical of lumbar dys-function. Although deep tendon reflexes and the straight leg raise (SLR) may be reduced (due to hamstring spasm), the clinical picture is usually one devoid of nerve root tension and other neurological signs (Mooney & Robertson, 1976; Kirkaldy-Willis & Hill, 1979; Fairbank *et al.*, 1981).

A recent paper by Helbig & Lee (1988) has suggested new diagnostic criteria for the lumbar facet syndrome in the form of a scorecard, having a total possible score of 100 points. This is the first time that an attempt has been made to weight factors involved in the criteria for the facet syndrome. This approach may well help to improve the accuracy of diagnosis as well as the predictability of treatment outcome.

Bernard & Kirkaldy-Willis (1988) have advocated the view that successful manipulative treatment confirms the diagnosis and identifies the contribution the posterior facets have had in the patient's current pain complex.

7.4 The sacro-iliac syndrome

There is little doubt that the sacroiliac syndrome has been a controversial topic for many years. The historical arguments have centred around, first, whether or not the joint is diarthrodial and, second, whether or not movement can occur (Greenman, 1986). Bowen & Cassidy (1981) have demonstrated that the sacro-iliac joint contains well developed cartilage surfaces, a synovial membrane, strong external ligaments and a large internal ligament. Numerous authors have described movements occurring in the sacro-iliac joints of cadavers and humans by means of various radiographic techniques (Weisl, 1954, 1955; Colochis *et al.*, 1963; Frigerio *et al.*, 1974; Egund *et al.*, 1978; Kirkaldy-Willis & Hill, 1979; Don Tigny, 1985). Chiropractors have supported the existence of both sacro-iliac dysfunction and the sacro-iliac syndrome, and have developed clinical tests for the detection of dysfunction of the joint (Gillet & Liekens, 1969; Gitelman, 1980). Recently a modified form these tests have been endorsed by a number of authors (Kirkaldy-Willis, 1983; Berg *et al.*, 1988).

The clinical picture of the sacro-iliac syndrome is well defined, although the mechanism of injury and the role the joint plays in the production of low back pain are not well understood (Kirkaldy-Willis & Hill, 1979). Some recent studies have attempted to address these problems. Berg *et al.* (1988) found that the most common cause of low back pain in women during pregnancy was sacro-iliac joint dysfunction.

The presenting complaint in the sacro-iliac syndrome is pain over one sacro-iliac joint in the region of the posterior superior iliac spine. The pain is usually described as dull in character and may be referred to the groin, anterior thigh or down the leg (Bernard & Kirkaldy-Willis, 1988). The pain is aggravated by sitting, arising from a chair, standing on the affected side and twisting (Gitelman, 1980).

Signs of the sacro-iliac syndrome include pain or tenderness to pressure over the involved sacro-iliac joint, dysfunction of movement in the joint, as detected by motion palpation tests and the absence of positive X-ray and neurological signs (Gitelman, 1980).

Whether one considers the sacro-iliac syndrome an extensor muscle and aponeurotic insertional strain syndrome, joint disorder, or a referred pain syndrome, there is little doubt that the large mechanical forces placed on the sacro-iliac joint during everyday activities may make this area a site of clinical pain (McGill, 1987).

7.5 Combined posterior facet and sacro-iliac joint syndrome

Bernard & Kirkaldy-Willis (1987) published a retrospective cohort study of 1293 cases of low back pain treated over a 12-year period at a university hospital low back pain clinic. Their findings indicated that sacro-iliac joint and posterior facet syndromes were the most common referred pain syndromes, whereas herniated nucleus pulposus and lateral nerve root entrapment were the most common nerve root compression syndromes. Of interest was the finding that referred pain syndrome were twice as common as radicular syndrome and that its clinical presentation may frequently mimic that of nerve root compression. More importantly, in nearly one-third of all patients there was more than one anatomical source of pain. Of these coexisting lesions, the most prevalent was the combination of posterior facet and sacro-iliac joint syndrome. A failure to recognise these lesions may lead to a less accurate diagnosis and poorer treatment response (Bernard & Kirkaldy-Willis, 1987).

7.6 Myofascial syndromes

Pain originating in the spine and related tissues such as the ligaments, joint capsule, outer portion of the annulus fibrosis and nerve root, as well as the patterns of pain distribution, have been described by numerous authors (Kellgren, 1939; Sunderland, 1975; Kellgren, 1977; McCall *et al.*, 1979; Yoshizawa *et al.*, 1980; Selby & Paris, 1981). Work by Simons & Travell (1983) and Travell & Simons (1984) has helped to elucidate the contribution of muscle in the genesis of low back pain. Myofascial syndromes can be important factors not only for the production of pain but also because of the similar referral patterns to the posterior facet syndrome, sacro-iliac joint syndrome, herniated nucleus pulposus and lateral spinal stenosis (Simons & Travell, 1983).

Six different syndromes, each implicating a different muscle, have been identified (see Table 7.2). The common features of the myofascial syndromes are local pain and tenderness at a characteristic site for each affected muscle (trigger point), referred pain often produced by pressure over the trigger point, again in a characteristic pattern, and a ropey or firm consistency around and including the trigger point (Kirkaldy-Willis, 1988). According to Bernard & Kirkaldy-Willis (1988), the diagnosis of a myofascial syndrome is made by physical findings and response to treatment by either anaesthetic or passive stretching.

Table 7.2   Myofascial syndromes

Gluteus maximus
Gluteus medius
Quadratus lumborum
Piriformis
Tensor fasciae latae
Hamstring

At present relatively little is known about the pathoanatomy and pathophysiology of the myofascial syndromes. What is apparent, however, is the importance of recognising a primary, secondary or coexisting myofascial lesion which may otherwise cloud the clinical picture of low back pain.

7.7 Summary

Any attempt to classify back pain syndromes is an immense task, as it is very difficult to produce an all-encompassing, all-inclusive system. Most classification systems have an author-generated bias. For these reasons, in this chapter no attempt has been made to provide an exhaustive list. There is no classification system that is universally accepted by the chiropractic profession. However, in terms of the direction in which chiropractic education is heading in the United Kingdom and Europe, the classification system presented is in step with current thought. The emphasis is directed towards chiropractors' perception of the most common back pain conditions.

In conclusion, classifications of back pain should perhaps be primarily based on simple clinical criteria that represents the majority of cases seen in clinical practice, as advocated by the Quebec Task Force on Spinal Disorders (Spitzer, 1987).

References

Arkin, A. M. (1950), The mechanism of rotation in combination with lateral deviation in the normal spine, *Journal of Bone and Joint Surgery*, **328**, 180–9.
Badgley, C. E. (1941), The articular facets in relation to low-back pain and sciatic radiation, *Journal of Bone and Joint Surgery*, **23**, 481–96.
Berg, G., Hammer, M., Moller-Nielsen, J., Linden, U. & Thorblad, J. (1988). Low back pain during pregnancy, *Obstetrics and Gynaecology*, **71**, 71–5.
Bernard, T. N. & Kirkaldy-Willis, W. H. (1987), Recognising specific characteristics of non-specific low back pain, *Clinical Orthopaedics*, **217**, 266–80.
Bernard, T. N. & Kirkaldy-Willis, W. H. (1988), Making a specific diagnosis. In: *Managing Low-Back Pain* (2nd Edn.) ed. W. H. Kirkaldy-Willis, pp. 209–27. Churchill-Livingstone, New York.
Bowen, V. & Cassidy, J. D. (1981), Macroscopic and microscopic anatomy of the sacroiliac joint from embryonic life until the eighth decade, *Spine*, **6**, 620–8.
Cassidy, J. D. (1976). Roentgenological examination of the functional mechanics of the lumbar spine in lateral flexion, *Journal of the Canadian Chiropractic Association*, July, 13–16.
Cassidy, J. D. & Potter, G. E. (1979), Motion examination of the lumbar spine, *Journal of Manipulative and Physiological Therapeutics*, **2**, 151.
Colochis, S. C., Warden, R. E., Bechtol, C. O. & Strohm, B. R. (1963), Movement of the sacro-iliac joint in the adult male: a preliminary report, *Archives of Physical Medicine and Rehabilitation*, **44**, 490–8.
Don Tigny, R. L. (1985), Function and pathomechanics of the sacro-iliac joint,

Physical Therapy, **65**, 35–44.

Dupuis, P. R., Yong-Hing, K., Cassidy, J. D. & Kirkaldy-Willis, W. H. (1985). Radiographic diagnosis of degenerative lumbar spinal instability, *Spine*, **10**, 262.

Egund, N., Alsson, T. H., Schmid, H. & Selvik, G. (1978), Movements in the sacro-iliac joints demonstrated with roentgen stereophotogrammetry, *Acta Radiologica: Diagnosis*, **19**, 833–46. i.

Fairbank, J. C. T., Park, W. M., McCall, I. W. & O'Brien, J. P. (1981), Apophyseal injection of local anaesthetic as a diagnostic aid in primary low-back syndromes, *Spine*, **6**, 598–605.

Frigerio, N. A., Stowe, R. R. & Howe, J. W. (1974), Movement of the sacro-iliac joint, *Clinical Orthopaedics and Related Research*, **100**, 370–7.

Frymoyer, J. W., Frymoyer, W. W., Wilder, D. G. & Pope, M. (1979), The mechanical and kinematic analysis of the lumbar spine in normal living human subjects *in vivo*, *Journal of Biomechanics*, **12**, 165.

Ghormley, R. K. (1933), Low-back pain with special reference to the articular facets, with presentation of an operative procedure, *Journal of the American Medical Association*, **101**, 1773–7.

Gillet, H. & Liekens, M. (1969), A further study of spinal fixations, *Annals of the Swiss Chiropractors' Association*, **4**, 41.

Gitelman, R. (1980), A chiropractic approach to biomechanical disorders of the lumbar spine and pelvis. In: *Modern Developments in the Principles and Practice of Chiropractic*, ed. S. haldeman, pp. 297–330. Appleton-Century-Crofts, Norwalk, Connecticut.

Goldthwait, J. E. (1911), The lumbosacral articulation: an explanation of many cases of lumbago, sciatica and paraplegia, *Boston Medical and Surgical Journal*, **164**, 365–72.

Greenman, P. E. (1986), Innominate shear dysfunction in the sacro-iliac syndrome, *Manual Medicine*, **2**, 114–21.

Gregersen, G. G. & Lucas, D. B. (1967), An *in vivo* study of axial rotation of the human thoracolumbar spine, *Journal of Bone and Joint Surgery*, **49A**, 247.

Grice, A. S. (1979), Radiographic, biomechanical and clinical factors in lumbar lateral flexion: Part 1, *Journal of Manipulative and Physiological Therapeutics*, **2**, 26.

Helbig, T. & Lee, C. K. (1988), The lumbar facet syndrome, *Spine*, **13**, 61–4.

Hirsch, C., Ingelmark, B. & Miller, M. (1963), The anatomical basis for low-back pain, *Acta Orthopaedica Scandinavica*, **33**, 1–17.

Kellgren, J. H. (1939), On the distribution of pain arising from deep somatic structures with charts of segmental pain areas, *Clinical Science*, **4**, 35–46.

Kellgren, J. H. (1977), The anatomical source of back pain, *Rheumatology and Rehabilitation*, **16**(1), 7–12.

King, J. S. & Lagger, R. (1976), Sciatica viewed as a referred pain syndrome, *Surgical Neurology*, **5**, 46–50.

Kirkaldy-Willis, W. H. (1983), The site and nature of the lesion. In: *Managing Low Back Pain*, (1st Edn.) ed. W. H. Kirkaldy-Willis, pp.91–107. Churchill-Livingstone, New York, Edinburgh, London, Melbourne.

Kirkaldy-Willis, W. H. (1988), The site and nature of the lesion. In: *Managing Low-Back Pain*, (2nd Edn.) ed. W. H. Kirkaldy-Willis, pp.138–41. Churchill-Livingstone, New York.

Kirkaldy-Willis, W. H. & Cassidy, J. D. (1985), Spinal manipulation in the treatment of low-back pain, *Canadian Family Physician*, **31**, 535–40.

Kirkaldy-Willis, W. H. & Hill, R. J. (1979), A more precise diagnosis for low-back pain, *Spine*, **4**, 102–9.

Lippit, A. B. (1984), The facet joint and its role in spine pain: management with facet joint injections, *Spine*, **9**, 746–50.

Lovett, R. W. (1905), The mechanism of the normal spine and its relation to scoliosis, *Boston Medical and Surgical Journal*, **153**, 349.

McCall, I. W., Park, W. M. & O'Brien, J. P. (1979), Induced pain referral from posterior lumbar elements in normal subjects, *Spine*, **4**, 441–6.

McGill, S. M. (1987), A biomechanical perspective of sacro-iliac pain, *Clinical Biomechanics*, **2**, 145–51.

Miles, M. & Sullivan, W. E. (1961), Lateral bending at the lumbar and lumbosacral joints, *Anatomical Record (New York)*, **139**, 387–98.

Mooney, V. & Roberson, J. (1976), The facet syndrome, *Clinical Orthopaedics*, **115**, 149–56.

Pearcy, M. J. & Tibrewal, S. B. (1984), Axial rotation and lateral bending in the normal lumbar spine measured by three-dimensional radiography, *Spine*, **9**, 582–7.

Selby, D. K. & Paris, S. V. (1981), Anatomy of facet joints and its correlation with lowback pain, *Contemporary Orthopaedics*, **312**, 1097–103.

Shealy, C. M. (1974), The role of the spinal facets in back and sciatic pain, *Headache*, **14**, 101–4.

Simons, D. G. & Travell, J. (1983), Myofascial origins of low-back pain: 1 principles of the diagnosis and treatment, *Postgraduate Medicine*, **73**, 99–108.

Spitzer, W. O. (Chairman) (1987), Scientific approach to the assessment and management of activity-related spinal disorders. A monograph for clinicians report of the Quebec Task Force on spinal disorders, *Spine*, **12**, S16-S21.

Sunderland, S. (1975), Anatomical perivertebral influences on the intervertebral foramen. In: *The Research Status of Manipulative Therapy*, pp. 129–40. NINCDS Monograph 15, US Department of Health Education and Welfare, Washington, DC

Travell, J. & Simons, D. G. (1984), Myofascial pain and dysfunction. In: *The Trigger Point Manual*, Williams & Wilkins, Baltimore.

Weisl, H. (1954), The articular surfaces of the sacroiliac joint and their relation to the movements of the sacrum, *Acta Anatomica*, **22**, 1–14.

Weisl, H. (1955), The movements of the sacroiliac joint, *Acta Anatomica*, **23**, 80–91.

Weitz, E. M. (1981), The lateral bending sign, *Spine*, **6**, 388–97.

Yoshizawa, H., O'Brien, J. P., Smith, W. T. & Trumper, M. (1980), The neuropathology of intervertebral discs removed for low-back pain, *Journal of Pathology*, **132**, 95–104.

Discussion

Fairbank: You have now introduced the concept of motion X-rays to the discussion. Many of us have doubts about the value of these X-rays. In studies where investigators have tried to look at their contribution to diagnosis, their reliability has been found to be poor. Could you perhaps comment on that?

Humphreys (in reply): I think we agree that static, non-motion X-rays are really of very little value in diagnosis of back pain. However, because we have a classification system which depends on the motion of the spine, we find that lateral bending stress X-rays seems to give us more information about the actual function of the spine than static films.

Fairbank: Do you have any reliability figures for this technique?

Humphreys (in reply): We are looking at spinal kinematics in two ways. One is by using a video-fluoroscopic digital-imaging process to assess spinal segmental movement incre-mentally (Breen, Robert & Morris, 1988; Breen *et al.*, 1989). The other involves gross intervertebral movement. The former technique is still at the calibration stage. For the latter, Cassidy (1976) showed that 25% of asymptomatic subjects showed abnormal distal wedging (Type III). We have shown (Bach, Lothe & Oestrich, 1988) that 100% of symptomatic subjects exhibited Type III motion on lateral bending.

Bach, L., Lothe, J. & Oestrich, A. (1988), A roentgenological study of the lumbar spine in lateral flexion in patients with low back pain, International Conference, *Spine and Low Back Pain Symposium*, Sydney.

Breen, A., Robert, A. & Morris, A. (1988). An Image processing method for spine kinematics, *Clinical Biomechanics*, **3**, 5–10.

Breen, A., Robert, A. & Morris, A. (1989). A digital videofluoroscopic technique for spine kinematics, *Journal of Biomedical Engineering*, **11**, 224–8.

Cassidy, J. D. (1976), Roentgenological examination of the functional mechanics of the lumbar spine in lateral flexion, *Journal of the Canadian Chiropractic Association*, July, 13–16.

The computer in syndromal diagnosis of low back disorders

8.1 Introduction

Low back pain and sciatica are the usual presenting symptoms of a wide variety of low back disorders. Syndromal diagnosis provides a clinical 'label' which is used for the management of the majority of patients seen in general practice, and for the referral and initial management of the minority of patients who require a structural diagnosis in the referral centre (Figure 8.1).

The important requirements in syndrome definition for decisions of management are not diagnostic but prognostic (Macartney, 1987). A syndrome 'label' poses the question: Will the prognostic benefits of making a precise structural diagnosis, with possible consequent treatment, outweigh the human and financial costs of obtaining that diagnosis? The decision to operate on any individual patient depends entirely on whether the surgeon can offer the patient a significantly more rapid and/or complete relief from disability than that associated with the natural history of the condition.

The clinician is faced with a wide variety of often ill-defined choices. For example, traditional medical methods (Huston, 1988; Wilson, 1988) are often less effective than clinical computing (Young, 1988; Mathew *et al.*, 1989) in ensuring the optimal utilisation of clinical information for patient management. All doctors are anxious not to miss a malignancy presenting as a low back disorder. Spinal surgeons have the added problem of the occasional negative exploration which can lead to the larger entity of 'the failed back syndrome' (Long *et al.*, 1988). In making these choices, clinicians may, inappropriately, ignore important indications or place too much emphasis on irrelevant or inaccurate information.

Most databases of patients illustrating these difficult questions in

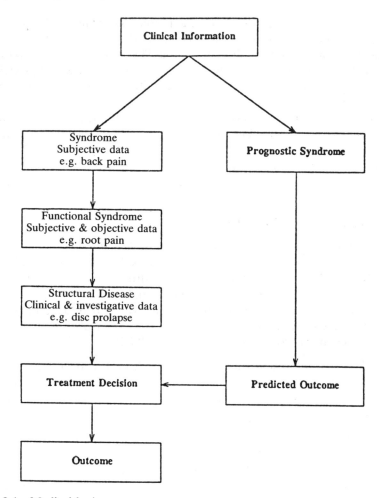

Fig. 8.1   Medical logic

medicine are small. The earlier pattern recognition techniques (*e.g.* Bayes's theorem) are imprecise in the mathematical modelling of data (Feinstein, 1977). Our system (CCAD) utilises a modern pattern recognition method which has performed well, even with small numbers of example patients, when optimal data modelling is crucial to diagnostic performance. In addition pattern recognition techniques allow objective analysis of clinical data, which can reveal the inherent syndromal patterns.

We have based our classification on a well documented and clinically validated approach (Waddell *et al.*, 1982, 1984; Morris *et al.*, 1986). So far we have looked at the clinical syndromes relevant to the differential diagnosis of low back disorders and the prediction of the likely operative findings in patients presenting with sciatica (Mathew *et al.*, 1988, 1989). As the management of low back disorders should be more related to prognosis than diagnosis, we are now in the process of using the same approach to search for prognostically related syndromes with respect to lumbar surgery (Figure 8.1).

If computerised pattern recognition continues to stand up to rigorous clinical scrutiny, then it has the potential to augment the structured assessment of patients in both community and hospital practice. This can rationalise both the investigation and treatment of these conditions and thus improve the usage of limited resources.

8.2 Defining the clinical problem

8.2.1 *Syndromes for differential diagnosis (i.e. Screening)*
Four functional syndromes have been defined (Nelson *et al.*, 1979; Waddell *et al.*, 1982/84; Uden *et al.*, 1988). These syndromes have both diagnostic and managerial implications. Although it might appear to be a trivial diagnostic task to categorise patients in this way, previous studies have shown that even experts can only achieve 80% inter-observer reliability and accuracy in this context (Waddell *et al.*, 1982).

(1) *Simple low back pain.* These patients have low back pain with or without referred thigh pain. Conservative management in the community is recommended for at least 3 months unless the clinical picture alters (Nachemson, 1980; Fager, 1984).

(2) *Root pain.* This group of patients have lumbar nerve root compression usually causing referred pain below the knee (*i.e.* sciatica). Some of these patients will require hospital treatment although the majority will recover spontaneously. The urgency of referral depends on the precise clinical findings (for example, sphincter involvement is a surgical emergency).

(3) *Spinal pathology.* This category includes patients with malignant, infective or inflammatory disorders. Diagnosis can be difficult and early investigation and treatment may alter prognosis (Cole, 1987; Blower, 1988; Francis *et al.*, 1988; Guyer *et al.*, 1988).

(4) *Abnormal illness behaviour.* This group of patients exhibit an exaggerated psychological response to their pain and disability. Routine referral is recommended to clinicians experienced in the evaluation and management of patients with a combination of organic and non-organic factors (Sternbach *et al.*, 1973; Waddell *et al.*, 1984).

It should be emphasised that patients may have one of the first three functional syndromes with or without abnormal illness behaviour. However, in the presence of psychological overlay it is difficult to interpret the clinical features. The fourth category has been defined to indicate the need for a more comprehensive assessment before functional classification is possible.

8.2.2 *Syndromes indicating operative findings in sciatica*

Three categories of operative findings have been defined and the clinical features identified for differentiating between them (Morris *et al.*, 1986; Mathew *et al.*, 1989).

(1) *No nerve root compression.* This includes patients who have a negative surgical exploration. No nerve root compression is found on either visual inspection or on passing a probe into the foramen.

(2) *Disc only and disc plus bony entrapment.* These patients have disc prolapse causing nerve root compression. Patients with combined disc and bony entrapment present with the same clinical picture.

(3) *Bony entrapment.* Surgical exploration reveals bony nerve root entrapment (i.e. lateral canal stenosis) without disc prolapse.

Patients with neurogenic claudication due to central canal stenosis were not included in this study. Inter-observer variation in surgical findings was minimised by independent observers and a formalised routine of eliciting and recording operative findings. However, it is not possible to eradicate inter-observer variation and this means that even surgical findings cannot be considered as a precise (reproducible) diagnostic end-point.

8.3 **Materials and methods**

8.3.1 *The computer system (CCAD)*

The computer (IBM PC) has been programmed to mimic the human ability to learn from example patients, termed inductive learning. The pattern recognition method is based in fuzzy logic (Norris *et al.*, 1986, 1987). This method is able to model the uncertainties and complexities found in biological systems, even when only small numbers of example patients are available, using discrimination and connectivity analyses. The discrimination approach effectively establishes a ranking of symptoms for their relative ability to distinguish between the diagnostic categories defined by subsequent specific structural diagnosis. The connectivity approach establishes which sets (i.e. clusters) of symptoms are particularly representative of each of the categories. Both these approaches are repeated positively and negatively, looking for symptoms that are or are not representative of each category.

CCAD has been validated on several different problems (Norris *et al.*, 1985, 1986; Mathew *et al.*, 1988, 1989) and against other methods of pattern recognition (Bounds *et al.*, 1988). CCAD can be applied to any medical problem that can be defined in terms of diagnostic outcomes, clinical features (i.e. symptoms, signs and investigations) and example patients.

CCAD learns by being presented with the clinical features of the

Table 8.1   Ranking tables computed as characteristic of the four general diagnostic categories (in decreasing order of importance)

Simple low back pain	Root pain
Night pain: no	Typical LMN pattern
Lumbar flexion > 5 cm	Involvement of 1 or 2 nerve roots
SLR limited by hamstrings	Sensory loss: yes
History of spinal fracture: yes	Positive myelogram
Structural scoliosis: yes	Loss of reflexes: yes
Thigh pain on drawing	Root pain on drawing
Walking makes bp worse: no	Motor loss: yes
Coughing makes bp worse: no	SLR limited by lp
Coughing makes lp worse: no	SLR ≤ 45°
Walking makes lp worse: no	sciatic list: yes
Age 20–55 yrs	Lp > bp
Caused by pregnancy	Site of pain: calf
Intolerance of treatments: yes	Coughing makes lp worse: yes
Dermatomal paraesthesia: no	Walking makes lp worse: yes
Duration: recurring	Site of pain: ankle

Spinal pathology	Abnormal illness behaviour
X-rays: true pathology	Whole leg giving way: yes
Non-mechanical bp	Increase slr on distraction: yes
ESR > 25 mm	Pain simulation axial load: yes
Acute duration ≤ 6 months	Non-anat tenderness: yes
Age ≥ 55	Over-reaction to examination: yes
Kyphosis: yes	Whole leg numbness: yes
Systemic symptoms: yes	Walking makes bp worse: yes
Other systemic diseases: yes	Pain simulation rotation: yes
Weight loss: yes	Intolerance of treatments: yes
History of carcinoma: yes	Non-anatomical pain drawing
Age ≤ 20 yrs	Source: problem referral
Onset: gradual	Very bizarre pain drawing
Site of pain: thoracic	Whole leg pain: yes
Typical UMN pattern	Never pain-free last year: yes
Whole leg giving way: no	Litigation involved: yes

Table 8.2   Ranking tables computed as characteristic of the three operative categories (in decreasing order of importance)

No root compression	Disc prolapse	Bony entrapment
Walking aggravates back/ upper leg pain	Definitive root irritation	SLR limited by hamstrings
Chronic root pain >12 months	Catch on straightening	No motor loss/minor sensory loss
Major problem = back/ upper leg pain	Sensory + motor loss	Generalised buttock and/or lumbar tenderness
Major problem = back pain	Early root pain ≤3 months	Root level = L5
No root pain	Muscle wasting	Subacute root pain ≤12 months
Pre-op disc criteria 0/4 or 1/4	Walking aggravates root pain	Pain score 0–30 mm
Walking causes sensory loss	Root level = L5 + S1	Walking aggravates root pain
Acute back problem ≤6 months	SLR limited by leg pain	SLR >75°/no root irritation
No root level	Pre-op disc criteria 3/4	Major problem = root pain
Back pain > leg pain	Major problem = root pain	Lumbar flexion >5 cm
Myelogram = none, normal or dural bulge	Myelogram = root cut-off + dural bulge	Myelogram = central stenosis or root cut-off
Doubtful root irritation	Crossed SLR +ve	Coughing has no effect on back/leg pain

example patients in each diagnostic category. This learning process provides a knowledge base against which a new patient's clinical features can be diagnosed. A ranking table of the specific clinical features calculated as being characteristic of each category is provided for empirical clinical analysis (Tables 8.1 and 8.2).

8.3.2 *Experimental method*
Differential diagnosis study (i.e. screening). Fifty patients from each of the four categories (i.e. 200 patients) were sequentially selected from a large patient database. The relevant clinical features had all been collected prospectively and recorded on a proforma. The patients had been followed up until the final structural diagnosis confirmed the original syndromal classification. In the category of spinal pathology there was missing clinical

information because some of these patients were very ill at the time of initial examination.

In each category the computer was used to produce a knowledge base from a 'training set' of 25 patients and then the other 25 ('test set') were diagnosed against this knowledge base by the computer. The 'test set' was then presented to a number of clinicians (i.e. family doctors, orthopaedic and neurosurgical registrars and consultants) who attempted to categorise them into the same four categories. The clinical information was then reduced to only the symptoms (i.e. contained in the clinical history) and the study repeated. All of the clinicians were aware that they were competing with a computer and had read two papers describing the clinical approach (Waddell *et al.*, 1982, 1984). In this way the diagnostic performance of the computer was compared to clinicians using varying amounts of clinical information.

CCAD was further tested in the differential diagnosis of 20 neurosurgical cases with conditions that were not included in the computer's knowledge base. These patients had either intradural lesions (i.e. cysts or benign/malignant tumours), thoracic disc prolapse or neurogenic claudication. Seventeen Bristol patients who had negative explorations for suspected disc prolapse were also analysed with this screening system.

Operative prediction study. This study consisted of 150 patients undergoing first time surgery for unilateral root pain (i.e. sciatica). All these patients' data were prospectively collected in Glasgow (90) and Bristol (60). For each patient the relevant clinical features (Mathew *et al.*, 1989; Kosteljanetz *et al.*, 1988) were recorded on a proforma.

Two pilot studies were done before arriving at a successful approach:

(1) The full set (i.e. including non-organic features) was used in the 'training set'. Also, combined disc and bony entrapment was inappropriately classified with bony entrapment alone.

Table 8.3 Comparison of percentage accuracy in differential diagnosis, the computer and six clinicians

	Simple low back pain	Root pain	Spinal pain	Abnormal illness b	Mean accuracy
Full assessment:					
Computer	100	92	80	88	90
Clinicians	85	90	70	80	83
Symptomatic assessment:					
Computer	60	92	80	96	82
Clinicians	70	70	70	78	70

(2) A human expert attempted to define for each operative category the classic symptoms, signs and investigative findings. When these were used as the 'training set' the computer could not diagnose satisfactorily.

The final and most successful approach was to reduce the clinical data-set by excluding non-organic symptoms and signs and reclassifying combined disc and bony entrapment with disc prolapse.

Six spinal surgeons (orthopaedic or neurosurgical registrars and consultants) were then tested in order to compare their accuracy in predictions to that of the computer. All of the surgeons were aware that they were competing with a computer and had read the paper which included a statistical analysis of the Glasgow patients (Morris *et al.*, 1986).

8.4 Results

The accuracy in diagnostic prediction is shown in Tables 8.3 and 8.4. CCAD out-performed the clinicians even though its patient knowledge base was relatively small. The system was robust in its ability to maintain

Table 8.4, Comparison of accuracy in operative prediction

	Glasgow patients			Bristol patients		
	No root	Disc	Bony	No root	Disc	Bony
Computer	92	75	68	62	78	64
BM	83	83	47	52	87	71
GW	75	68	5	67	78	36
CM	83	65	0	52	74	29
AR	92	70	21	62	74	29
DA	75	62	63	52	74	57
TR	50	75	32	38	74	43

Table 8.5 False positives and negatives for operative prediction

	Glasgow patients		Bristol patients	
	False positives	False negatives	False positives	False negatives
Computer	1	10	14	5
BM	2	13	17	2
GW	3	29	12	14
CM	2	31	17	17
AR	1	27	14	15
DA	3	15	17	5
TR	7	15	22	10

accuracy in diagnosis in spite of incomplete data and heterogeneous patients from different centres and surgical disciplines. False positives and negatives were kept to a minimum (Table 8.5) and were all found to give good interpretations of available clinical data with uncertainty reflected where it was indicated. It is important to emphasise that whilst the CCAD diagnosis was not infallible, it was nevertheless more accurate than any of the clinicians.

During CCAD's learning process, a profile of each disease was calculated from the patient data in the 'training set'. These ranking tables are shown in Tables 8.1 and 8.2. For the sake of simplicity we have only shown the positive criteria that support a particular diagnosis. The importance of the symptomatic history is shown by the prominence of symptoms in these ranking tables. The profile calculated as characteristic of each category is in accord with empiric clinical observation by human experts (Dixon, 1980; Wynn Parry et al., 1988). However, when the expert attempted to construct a knowledge base without using example patient data, this did not prove reliable for computerised diagnosis.

Non-organic signs were shown to be more specific than non-organic symptoms in accurately identifying abnormal illness behaviour. Non-organic symptoms proved too sensitive as they gave many false positives. This is why the computer was more accurate than the clinicians in diagnosing simple low back pain (symtomatic assessment). In the operative prediction study, non-organic symptoms and signs appeared to reduce diagnostic accuracy. These were more prevalent in the bony compression category in Glasgow and in the no root compression category in Bristol, thus confusing diagnosis between the two centres.

Eight of the 17 Bristol patients who subsequently had negative explorations for suspected disc prolapse were diagnosed (CCAD screening version) as having abnormal illness behaviour. Knowing this might have avoided unnecessary surgery and indicates that psychological overlay cannot be dismissed in managerial decision making.

In differential diagnosis (i.e. screening) the family doctors were virtually equal to the surgeons in diagnostic accuracy. In operative prediction the surgeons had few false positives. This is important as unnecessary surgical exploration is best avoided. There was a marked difference in individual surgeons ability to predict operative findings. They had all read the paper describing the Glasgow series (Morris et al., 1986) and this identifies the fact that bony entrapment is frequently associated with few clinical signs. In spite of having just read this paper, false negatives (i.e. missing surgically treatable lesions) were most prominent in patients with bony entrapment (Kirkaldy Willis et al., 1982).

The surgeons' tendency to overlook patients with minimal signs may reflect their anticipation of a less satisfactory surgical outcome. The 20 false negative patients in the Glasgow series (i.e. diagnosed by the surgeons as no root compression but found at surgery to have it) were followed up carefully. Of the 11 patients with disc prolapse, ten did extremely well post operatively. However, only three of the nine with bony entrapment did well following surgery. Therefore, in this study, surgery was more successful in disc prolapse than in bony entrapment when minimal signs were present.

The differential diagnosis system was used on 20 neurosurgical patients with disorders not included in the CCAD knowledge base. Intradural lesions (i.e. arachnoid cysts, benign and malignant tumours) and thoracic disc prolapse were classified by computer as spinal pathology. However, when only symptoms were considered these patients tended to be misclassified as abnormal illness behaviour. Neurogenic claudication was classified as root pain. CCAD requires the addition of several diagnostic categories and corresponding example patients. These categories include spinal deformities, rheumatological conditions, neurogenic claudication and neurological disorders. This is being undertaken at present.

8.5 Discussion

The lack of conformity in the surgeons' prediction of operative findings, having just read the same paper (Morris *et al.*, 1986), illustrates the difficulty in improving diagnostic performance by traditional educational means (Huston, 1988; Wilson, 1988). By contrast, computerised pattern recognition has the potential to provide an objective evaluation of the diagnostic process thus identifying optimal diagnostic logic. This will serve to improve communication between doctors by reducing diagnostic idiosyncrasy thus enabling the rationalisation of patient management. The most useful areas of clinical application will be those which doctors find most difficult. Screening of large numbers of symptomatic patients, behavioural assessment and prognostic prediction are suitable examples.

Clinical complacency engendered by 'yet another backache' can lead to failure in diagnosing the few patients with underlying serious pathology. Early diagnosis can be difficult and is known to effect prognosis (Cole, 1987; Blower, 1988; Francis *et al.*, 1988; Guyer *et al.*, 1988). CCAD (screening) has demonstrated its potential to aid doctors in this difficult area of diagnosis.

In spinal surgery the common belief is that unequivocal lumbar nerve entrapment by either disc prolapse or lateral canal stenosis is associated with a good prognosis and a negative exploration with a poor prognosis (Spangforth, 1972; Getty, 1980; Long *et al.*, 1988). Bony entrapment is difficult to diagnose both pre-operatively and at surgery (Kirkaldy Willis *et al.*, 1982). In consequence CCAD has the potential to improve both specificity and sensitivity of surgical intervention. Unnecessary and possibly harmful surgery can be prevented by predicting the likelihood of a negative exploration. Bony entrapment is less likely to be missed due to improved diagnostic sensitivity. The discrimination of disc prolapse from bony nerve root entrapment allows the appropriate choice of treatment.

Prognosis remains the most important consideration. Irrespective of structural diagnosis it is vital to operate only on those patients who will really benefit. If prognostically related syndromes (i.e. based on observational data alone) can be found for lumbar surgery then these can be used for triage in the large (community-based) symptomatic population. Surgical priorities can be established based on an objective measure of those patients who will benefit maximally.

While CCAD will not replace doctors (Pringle, 1988) it can provide a 'tunable' management grid, based on observational (i.e. no expensive investigations) clinical information. The system can be custom-built to the specific needs of each practice. This technology can improve patient management by both rigorous data collection and analysis, and automation of secretarial tasks including clinical audit.

Acknowledgements

The authors wish to thank their neurosurgical and orthopaedic colleagues in Bristol and Glasgow for collecting and analysing data. Tables 8.2, 8.4, and 8.5 have been reproduced with permission from the *British Journal of Neurosurgery*.

References

Blower, P. W. (1988), Backpain at Greenwich, *Journal of the Royal Society of Medicine*, **81**, 203–6.

Bounds, D. G., Lloyd, P. J., Mathew, B. G. & Waddell, G. (1988), A multilayer perceptron network for the diagnosis of low back pain, *Proceedings of the 2nd International Conference in Neural Networks*, Santiago, Illinois, pp. 481–7.

Cole, R. P. (1987), Low back pain and testicular cancer, *British Medical Journal*, **295**, 840–1.

Dixon, A. St J. (1980), Diagnosis of low back pain, *The Lumbar Spine and Back Pain* (2nd Edn.), pp. 135–55, Pitman Publishers, London.

Fager, C. A. (1984), The age-old back problem, *Spine*, **9**, 326–8.

Feinstein, A. R. (1977), Clinical biostatistics XXIV: The haze of Bayes', the aerial palaces of decision analysis and the computerised ouija board, *Clinical Pharmacological Therapeutics*, **21**, 482–96.

Francis, N. D., Das, S., Tyrrell, P. (1988), Osteomyelitis with rapidly fatal course, *Journal of the Royal Society of Medicine*, **81**, 51–2.

Getty, C. J. M. (1980), Lumbar spinal stenosis: The clinical spectrum and results of operations, *Journal of Bone and Joint Surgery*, **62**, 481–5.

Guyer, R. D., Collier, R. R., Ohnmeiss, D. D., Stith, W. J., Hochschuler, S. H., Rashbaum, R. F., Vanharanta, H. & Loguidice, V. (1988), Extraosseous spinal lesions mimicking disc disease, *Spine*, **13**, 328–31.

Huston, G. J. (1988), An offer of rheumatology training: failure to influence clinic referrals, *British Medical Journal*, **296**, 1773–4.

Kirkaldy Willis, W. H., Wedge, J. H. & Yong Hing, A. (1982), Lumbar spine nerve lateral entrapment, *Clinical Orthopaedics*, **169**, 171–8.

Kosteljanetz, M., Bang, F. & Schmidt-Olsen, S. (1988), The clinical significance of straight-leg raising in the diagnosis of prolapsed lumbar disc: Interobserver variation and correlation with surgical findings, *Spine*, **13**, 393–5.

Long, D. M., Filtzer, D. L., Ben Debba, M. & Hendler, N. H. (1988), Clinical features of the failed back syndrome, *Journal of Neurosurgery*, **69**, 61–71.

McCartney, F. J. (1987), Diagnostic logic, *British Medical Journal*, **295**, 1325–31.

Mathew, B. G., Norris, D. E., Hendry, D. & Waddell, G. (1988), Artificial Intelligence in the diagnosis of low back pain and sciatica, *Spine*, **13**, 168–72.

Mathew, B. G., Norris, D. E., Mackintosh, I. & Waddell, G. (1989), Artificial Intelligence in the prediction of operative findings in low back surgery, *British Journal of Neurosurgery*, **3**, 161–70.

Morris, E. W., Di Paola, M., Vallance, R. & Waddell, G. (1986), Diagnosis and decision making in lumbar disc prolapse and nerve entrapment, *Spine*, **11**, 436–9.

Nachemson, A. (1980), A critical look at conservative treatment for low back pain. In: *The lumbar spine and back pain* (2nd Edn.), pp. 453–66, Pitman Publishers, London.

Nelson, M. A., Allen, P., Clamp, S. E. & De Dombal, F. T. (1979), Reliability and reproducibility of clinical findings in low back pain *Spine*, **4**, 97–101.

Norris, D. E. (1986), Machine learning using fuzzy logic with applications in medicine, PhD Thesis, University of Bristol, England.

Norris, D. E., Jones, R., Mathew, B. G. & Pilsworth, B. (1985), Development aspects of computer aided diagnosis, *Bristol Medical Chirurgical Journal*, **100**, 376, 101–5.

Norris, D. E., Pilsworth, B. W. & Baldwin, J. F. (1987), Medical diagnosis from patients records: A method using fuzzy discrimination and connectivity analyses, *Fuzzy Sets and Systems*, **23**, 73–88.

Pringle, M. (1988), Using computers to take patient histories, *British Medical Journal*, **297**, 697.

Spangforth, E. V. (1972), The lumbar disc herniation: a computer-aided analysis of 2504 operations, *Acta Orthopaedica Scandinavia*, (suppl.) 142, S1–S95.

Sternbach, R. A., Wolf, S. R., Murphy, R. W. & Akeson, W. M. (1973), Traits of pain patients: The low-back 'loser', *Psychosomatics*, **14**, 226–29.

Uden, A., Astrom, M. & Bergenudd, H. (1988), Pain drawings in chronic back pain, *Spine*, **13**, 389–92.

Waddell, G., Bircher, M., Finlayson, D. & Main, C. J. (1984), Symptoms and signs: Physical disease or illness behaviour, *British Medical Journal*, **289**, 739–41.

Waddell, G., Main, C. J., Morris, F. W., Venner, R. M., Rae, P. S., Sharmy, S. H. & Galloway, H. (1982), Normality and reliability in clinical assessment of backache, *British Medical Journal*, **284**, 1519–23.

Wilson, D. G. (1988), The invaluable art of unlearning, *Journal of the Royal Society of Medicine*, **81**, 3–6.

Wynn Parry, C. B., Girgis, F., Morfat, B. & Bhalla, A. K. (1988), The failed back: a review, *Journal of the Royal Society of Medicine*, **81**, 348–51.

Young, D. W. (1988), Numerical methods for decision-making in clinical care: Where to now? *Journal of the Royal Society of Medicine*, **81**, 128–9.

Discussion

Fairbank: Are you suggesting that the non-organic signs and symptoms are non-contributory or reverse contributory on arriving at these diagnoses?

Mathew (in reply): No, I think they are contributory. Negative surgical explorations in patients with marked illness behaviour were more common in Bristol than Glasgow. This is probably explained by the Glasgow group's interest in non-organic features. So, they are useful but one has to be careful that they are not misunderstood. The presence of non-organic features may influence patient management but does not exclude the possibility of treatable organic pathology.

Nelson: Your outcome measure, the response to surgery, requires close scrutiny. We know from the work of Weber, for example, that most people with severe disc prolapses get better in time and it is quite clear from a neurosurgical paper in *The Lancet* some while ago (Thomas *et al.*, 1983) that if you operate on everybody very early you do get very good results, perhaps because many of the people did not need surgery at all. Even if you find a disc prolapse at operation, we know that there is plenty of evidence to show that when the patient recovers, the filling defect can still be seen on a myelogram. So, even surgical assessment, unfortunately, has to be questioned in this type of analysis.

Weber, H. (1983), Lumbar disc herniation A controlled, prospective study with ten years of observation, *Spine*, **8**, 131–140.
Thomas, M., Grant, N., Marshall, J. & Stevens, J. (1983), Surgical treatment of low backache and sciatica, *Lancet*, **ii**, 1437–9.

Mathew (in reply): If you, in fact, build your net from patients who you have operated on and made worse ...

Nelson: That does not work you see, because I am still saying that these patients could get better if you waited long enough and the fact that you operated on them does not mean that you needed to operate on them.

Mathew (in reply): How long do you wait? Surgeons are operating on disc prolapse in an effort to reduce the duration of disability. No optimal time for intervention has been established. However, surgery should definitely be avoided in patients likely to have a negative exploration and those whose symptoms are likely to be unchanged or worse post operatively. This is what we are looking at.

Eisenstein: I have this feeling as the morning progresses we have Kipling's elephant. Often we are feeling different parts of it, and even if we feel the same part, we have different interpretations about what we are feeling. Bruce Mathew and I have spoken about this before. You speak as though it is quite settled, for example, as to what the non-organic symptoms and signs are. I would like to suggest that is not so, despite various statistics and studies. This is such a highly personal area that I wonder if we are ever going to develop a co-ordinated approach.

Mathew (in reply): My emphasis here, and indeed my contribution, has been the concept of pattern recognition. I would put it to you that you can use any classification you wish and teach a computer using your own patient database, a group of related symptoms and signs, and outcomes. The system will probably out-perform you in classifying new patients because it provides an objective method of 'pattern matching'. This allows you to use the computer to assess a new patient with respect to your own experience.

Sweetman: Can I take you up on that last point. What are you using as your ulti-mate truth? With the first group you had the training set and the test set, and you say that the computer wins every time. Is that because it is making up the rules as it goes along? It says, 'I have got this right', while we as the clinicians are trying to imitate what the computer does. Obviously the computer does better. Yet if we say that everything we say is right, the computer does not do as well as us, if you take the clinicians' prediction of diagnostic group as the ultimate criterion of success. How are you defining your ultimate truth of diagnosis in the test set?

Mathew (in reply): The outcome has been carefully determined before the start of the study (see 8.3.2). The problem you describe will occur when such systems are introduced into daily practice. Initial blinded trials can avoid such 'feed-back arte-fact'. The actual prognostic outcome will probably prove the most reproducible, objective endpoint against which to measure predictive accuracy.

Jayson: Could you tell us what 'Fuzzy Logic' is?

Mathew (in reply): It essentially establishes any fact between 0 and 1 (i.e. no = 0, yes = 1). You might define 'maybe' as 0.3 and 'probably' as 0.7 on this scale. So it is an attempt to model uncertainty.

Sweetman: Is that any different for setting your mean to 0 and your standard devia-tion to 1, which is the basis of many of the cluster techniques?

Mathew (in reply): CCAD uses connected sets which are similar to cluster analysis (see Norris *et al.*, 1987 for numerical aspects). When we used other methods of pattern recognition (Bounds *et al.*, 1988) they all performed quite well so I am not saying that our method is the only one. The important thing is to model the inter-relatedness of the clinical features by not assuming independence (i.e. Bayes' theorem). Clearly symptoms and signs are inter-related (i.e. clustered) in most clinical problems.

Bounds, D. G., Lloyd, P. J., Mathew, B. G. & Waddell, G. (1988), A multi layer perceptron network for the diagnosis of low back pain, *Proceedings of the 2nd International Conference in Neural Networks*, Santiago, Illinois, pp. 481–7.

Norris, D. E., Pilsworth, B. W. & Baldwin, J. F. (1987), Medical diagnosis from patients records: A method using fuzzy discrimination and connectivity analyses, *Fuzzy Sets and Systems*, **23**, 73–88.

Mulholland: Retuning to the issue of the validity of the presence or absence of a disc protrusion. There appeared to be a number of patients who were operated on for disc protrusion when they had all the clinical symptoms, but the myelogram was essentially normal, or absent. So it seems as if the surgeon was attaching greater value to his clinical judgement and ignoring the investigation. How did the com-puter handle that? The computer presumably would predict that no disc protrusion would be found at surgery.

Mathew (in reply): Occasionally patients were operated on in spite of normal myelogram findings because it was felt that they had lateral bony root entrapment which is not always visualised by myelogram. The patients who did not have myelo-grams had CAT scans. The computer's prediction of likely operative findings was based more on clinical features than radiological appearance (Table 8.2). This is why its diagnostic predictions remain pretty accurate in spite of false positive, false negative or absent radiology.

The relationship of developmental spinal canal stenosis to vertebral and skeletal morphology

9.1 Introduction

Degenerative spine disease is common (Lawrence *et al.*, 1963) and can result in severe disability and pain. It is generally appreciated that where there is already pre-existing narrowing (i.e. developmental stenosis) of the spinal canal then the clinical features may be more severe and may occur with relatively little degenerative disease (Payne & Spillane, 1957; Hinck & Sachdev, 1966; Nurick, 1972; Epstein *et al.*, 1977). Although the factors responsible for degenerative disease have been extensively studied, the pathogenesis of developmental spinal canal stenosis has not. One possible explanation is that canal size is related to overall skeletal size, but it is not the experience of most clinicians that the canals of large people are capacious, nor that those of small people are stenotic. If not related to overall skeletal size, could canal dimensions be associated with particular body shape or somatotype? Similarly could canal size be related to vertebral shape rather than overall vertebral size?

A possible association between somatotype and canal size is suggested from two sources. Firstly, in achondroplasia, an autosomal dominant condition in which a particular somatotype is characterised by short long bones and relatively normal size of head and trunk, the subjects also have very narrow canals mainly due to shortening of the pedicles which themselves grow in the manner of long bones (Lutter, 1978). By analogy with achondroplasia, one might expect that in those with idiopathic canal stenosis, short pedicles might be associated with short long bones elsewhere. Indeed the possibility that canal stenosis is a *forme fruste* of achondroplasia has been considered (Roberts, 1978). A second possible association of somatotype and canal size arises from anthropological studies between different racial groups. For example, among the North African Nilotic tribes somatotype is strikingly slender with relatively long limbs compared to trunk length, whereas the Mongoloid races are more stocky with relatively short limbs compared to trunk length. The observation that different racial groups tend to have canals of different sizes (Eisenstein, 1976; Postacchini *et al.*, 1983) suggests a possible genetic association between somatotype and canal size. In the literature concerning vertebral canal stenosis, there are a few comments that suggest that the possibility of such an association between somatotype and canal size has been considered. Most discount this possibility (Verbiest, 1975, 1976, 1980; Weinstein, 1980). However, McRae (1977) has commented that 'thickset individuals' tend to develop lumbar canal stenosis and Babin (1980) states: 'It is notable that the anteroposterior diameter varies always with biotype, race and with the more or less important muscular strains in professional and sportive activities'. However, in none of these references, either those for or against a possible association, are data provided to substantiate these statements nor is a reference to previously published anthropometric studies provided.

The relationship of developmental stenosis to vertebral size and shape has not been systematically studied, but some radiologists have suggested that these patients may have particular abnormalities on their lumbar spine X-rays. Commonly quoted radiological features are listed in Table 9.1; the claims for each individual feature are discussed in more detail elsewhere (Nightingale, 1986). Most proponents of these X-ray features consider only one in isolation and no study of their inter-relationship has been attempted. For example, one does not know if these various features account for the same variation in developmental canal size or whether they are independent of one another.

The aim of this study is to investigate the relationship of developmental

Table 9.1   Radiographic features reported to be abnormal in lumbar canal stenosis

---

Interpedicular distance
Pedicle thickness
Visibility of posterior intervertebral joints
Angulation of posterior intervertebral joints
Height of posterior intervertebral joints
Proximity of posterior intervertebral joints
Apophyso-vertebral ratio
Interlaminar space dimensions
Interlaminar space asymmetry
Pedicle length
Pedicle thickness
Intervertebral foramen dimensions
Vertebral body dimensions

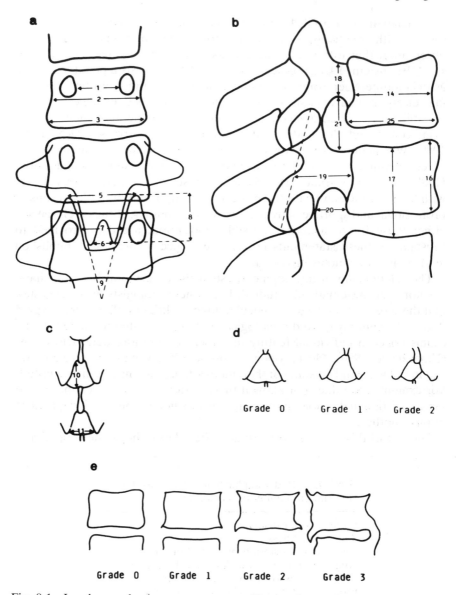

Fig. 9.1 Lumbosacral spine measurements. The numbers refer to measurements described in the text. (a) AP projection; (b) lateral projection; (c) interlaminar space asymmetry; (e) osteophytosis

spinal canal stenosis firstly to the shape of the vertebra and secondly to that of the skeleton.

9.2 **Methods**

One hundred and two patients were studied, all aged over 18 by which time the relative proportions of the skeletal components have become fixed. The measure of developmental canal size was taken as the AP diameter of the radio-opaque theca opposite the waist of the vertebral body at the narrowest part, most commonly opposite the body of L3 or L4. In the cervical region developmental canal size was measured on plain lateral projection radiographs and taken as the AP diameter of the spinal canal at the C6 vertebral body from the midpoint of the posterior surface of the vertebral body to the nearest part of the line formed by the junction of the laminae. The assessment of vertebral shape was made using the following measurements taken at each of the five lumbar vertebral levels or at the next caudal intervertebral level (Figure 9.1).

On the AP projection:

(1) interpedicular distance

(2) side-to-side vertebral body width at the waist

(3) side-to-side vertebral body width at the lower margin, excluding osteophytes

(4) visibility of the two posterior intervertebral joints. This was recorded as: 0 when one or both were not visible; 1 when both could be seen sufficiently well for the measurements to be made, but not very clearly; 2 when both were seen very clearly

(5) distance between the tips of the superior facets of the posterior intervertebral joints

(6) distance between the tips of the inferior facets of the posterior intervertebral joints

(7) distance between the radiolucent posterior intervertebral joints at the level of the pedicles

(8) height of the posterior intervertebral joint in a craniocaudal direction

(9) the acute angle created by extrapolating the lines formed by joining the cranial and caudal ends of the posterior intervertebral joints using a transparent plastic goniometer

(10) the craniocaudal height of the radiolucent area formed between the caudal margin of one lamina and the cranial margin of the lamina below (the 'interlaminar space')

(11) the side-to-side dimension of the interlaminar space

(12) the degree of irregularity and asymmetry of the interlaminar space. This was recorded as: 0 when there was no asymmetry; 1 with mild asymmetry; 2 with marked asymmetry

(13) the degree of osteophytosis of the vertebral bodies was graded by the criteria of Eisenstein (1977). This was recorded as: 0 where no osteophytes were apparent; 1 when there were mild osteophytes; 2 with moderate osteophytes; 3 with severe osteophytes.

On the lateral projection:

(14) AP vertebral body width at the waist

(15) AP vertebral body width at the lower margin, excluding osteophytes

(16) vertebral body craniocaudal height

(17) disc space height

(18) craniocaudal thickness of the pedicle

(19) Eisenstein's measure of the AP canal size (Eisenstein, 1977)

(20) the AP dimension of the intervertebral foramen from the posterior surface of the vertebral body to the anterior surface of the inferior facet, excluding osteophytes

(21) the craniocaudal dimension of the intervertebral foramen

(22) the AP dimension of the whole vertebra from the anterior surface of the vertebral body at the waist to the posterior limit of the spinous process.

Both the cervical and lumbar measurements were corrected for magnification. The former by the use of a radio-opaque marker and the latter by a correction factor derived for each patient based on pelvic measurements. The further details of these calculations and discussion of the importance of correction for magnification is provided elsewhere (Nightingale, 1986). Skeletal morphology (i.e. somatotype) was assessed in 91 subjects (65 men, 26 women) using standard anthropometric techniques (Cameron, 1978). Standing and sitting height were measured using a Harpenden stadiometer. Foot, tibia, upper arm and lower arm lengths, bicondylar femur and humerus diameters, bi-iliocristal and bi-acromial diameters were obtained using a Harpenden anthropometer. Head and chest circumference was obtained using a tapemeasure and weight by using a balance weighing machine.

9.3 **Results**

9.3.1 *Vertebral morphology and canal size*

Of all the many different measurements a number showed a significant correlation with lumbar canal size. The inter-relationship of these various features can be studied in several ways. For example, each variable in turn can be correlated with each of the others in turn resulting in a large correlation matrix. Alternatively one can mathematically transform these variables, using principal component analysis (Kim, 1983), into a new set of variables that account for the same overall variation but in which the first transformed variable or component accounts for the maximum overall variation among the original standardised variables, the second component for the maximum residual variation independent of the first and so forth. The first three components produced in this way (Table 9.2) accounted for over two-thirds of the variation and roughly divided the variables into three independent groups. In the first component are pedicle thickness, facet joint height and vertebral body diameter. In the second are width of the intervertebral foramen, interlaminar space width and Eisenstein's measure. The third component loads mainly for the visibility of the facet joint on the AP films reflecting its more saggital orientation in those with narrow canals. Much of the unexplained variation is probably related to either measurement error or some source of variation unique to individual variables. This sort of analysis demonstrates that these variables are not merely different measures of the same thing – such as overall vertebral

Table 9.2   Principal component analysis of lumbar spine measurements. The variable numbers refer to measurements described in the methods section

Variable	Component 1	Component 2	Component 3
1	0.44	0.57	0.06
2	0.87	0.05	0.12
4	−0.51	−0.05	0.81
8	0.77	−0.04	−0.04
11	0.00	0.85	−0.22
14	0.89	0.04	0.01
16	0.38	0.03	0.59
18	0.77	0.08	0.12
19	0.07	0.67	0.59
20	−0.31	0.69	0.11

Table 9.3   Multiple regression analysis of lumbar spine measurements.
The variable numbers refer to measurements described in the methods section:
$r = 0.72$; $r^2 = 0.52$; SEE = 1.34 mm

Variable	B	SEB	BETA	p
18	−0.58	0.16	−0.40	0.005
19	0.23	0.10	0.26	0.02
1	0.02	0.75	0.28	0.01
11	0.08	0.31	0.26	0.009
14	−0.15	0.66	−0.25	0.02
Constant	12.47	2.65		<0.001

size, but that the vertebral shape itself can be assessed and described by this analysis. It also means that these variables can be combined in a multiple regression equation to predict canal size more accurately than an equation using one variable alone. Various regression models can be derived depending on which combination of variables is chosen. A typical model is shown in Table 9.3. The regression model was obtained using 'stepwise' analysis (Nie *et al.*, 1983). B represents the partial regression coefficient and SEB is the standard error of B. The named independent variables (VAR) are listed in the order of stepwise selection. BETA, the standardised partial regression coefficient, provides a better comparison of the coefficients when the variables differ markedly in magnitude or are measured in different units. The important summary statistics are firstly the correlation coefficient (r) between the predicted canal size and the actual canal size; secondly r^2 which here is 0.52 indicating that over 50% of the variation in canal size can be accounted for by the regression model; and thirdly the standard error of the estimate which means that approximately 68% of individuals will have an actual size within 1.3 mm of the predicted canal size. A regression model is generally better at predicting the dependent variable in the data from which it is derived than from an independent sample. The model was therefore tested by dividing the data into two halves. On one half the regression model was derived and then tested on the other half. For the regression equation provided in Table 9.3, this resulted in an r^2 of 0.46, only a modest reduction from 0.52. Further details of the statistical analysis of the relationship of canal size to vertebral morphology using multivariate analysis and several alternative regression models can be found elsewhere (Nightingale, 1986).

9.3.2 *Relationship of somatotype to canal size*
To study the inter-relationship of the anthropometric variables, factor analysis was performed using 'principle factoring' with an iteration pro-

cedure for improving the estimates of communalities (Kim, 1983). Two factors accounted for 76% of the total variance of the original data and VARIMAX rotation to a terminal solution produced a first factor that loaded mainly on ectomorphic variables such as height and limb length and a second factor loading mainly for endomorphic variables such as weight, chest circumference, etc. Knee and elbow size, head circumference and biochromial diameter loaded on both factors. A third factor with an Eigenvalue of 0.95 loaded primarily on knee width, head circumference and sitting height (Table 9.4). The relationship of somatotype to canal size was determined in two ways. Firstly multiple regression analysis (Table 9.5) showed that there was a significant association of cervical canal size with subjects whose trunk was long as measured by their sitting height but who had reduced long bone length in particular the upper arm. Regression analysis showed that although the model was statistically significant it only accounted for 22% of the variation in cervical canal size. No significant equation of this kind could be derived from the lumbar canal. The second method of relating somatotype to canal size was by visual inspection of the superimposed somatotype standardised pattern profiles of subjects with

Table 9.4   Factor analysis of somatotype variables

Variables	Factor 1	Factor 2	Factor 3
Foot length	0.69	0.29	0.35
Tibial length	0.82	0.40	−0.01
Knee diameter	0.51	0.46	0.56
Bicristal diameter	0.28	0.55	0.32
Biacromial diameter	0.39	0.55	0.15
Upper arm length	0.66	0.20	0.16
Lower arm length	0.71	0.36	0.02
Elbow diameter	0.47	0.36	0.38
Head circumference	0.06	0.24	0.55
Chest circumference	0.15	0.94	0.23
Weight	0.40	0.81	0.34
Sitting height	0.64	0.06	0.45
Height	0.90	0.20	0.29

Table 9.5   Multiple regression analysis of somatotype variables. $r = 0.47$; $r^2 = 0.22$; SEE = 10.4

Variable	B	SEB	BETA	*p*
Upper arm length	0.31	0.06	0.55	<0.0001
Sitting height	−0.05	0.02	−0.25	0.03
Constant	95.2	21.2		<0.0001

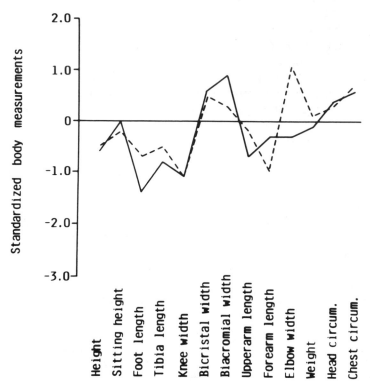

Fig. 9.2 Standardised somatotype pattern profiles of two subjects to show similarity of somatotype

narrow canals to try and detect somatotypes in common. Examples shown in Figure 9.2 supported the results of the multiple regression analysis.

9.4 Discussion

It is clear from these results that developmental canal stenosis is not an isolated skeletal anomaly. Although much is known about overall skeletal growth *in utero* and postnatally, little is known about the factors that control the relative growth of bones in different parts of the body. It is possible that, in those with canal stenosis, some environmental factor has influenced both the development of the canal and growth of various parts of the vertebra and skeleton at some critical stage. It is however more likely that the association of canal stenosis with the vertebral shape and somatotype is inherited. The numerous publications over the last few decades suggest an interest in predicting developmental spinal canal size in the lumbar region from plain film measurements. The multivariate analyses described above and elsewhere (Nightingale, 1986) have demonstrated that combining measurements in a linear equation allows estimation of the developmental canal narrowing with a reasonable accuracy. The variables may be combined effectively in various ways since they account in different proportions for the various factors that determine canal size. In this way, it is possible for the radiologist to assess the extent of developmental canal stenosis on the plain film radiographs by specifically looking at those features that correlate with canal size.

In general, the more of these features that are abnormal and the greater the degree of the abnormality, then the narrower will be the canal. However, principal component analysis and multiple regression equations have shown that some features account for the same variation in canal size. For these features, the finding of several correlated abnormalities provides no better prediction than finding a single abnormality. Nevertheless, if all such features are abnormal, then an error of radiological measurement is less likely and a choice of radiological feature to examine may be helpful if the radiograph is indistinct. On the other hand, the multivariate analyses have shown that some radiographic features are independently related to canal size, so that the finding of more than one abnormality may be much more significant than finding only one. For example, the observation of abnormalities of both interlaminar space width and posterior intervertebral joint height is a better predictor of canal stenosis than that of either alone.

Based on the results outlined above, a simple method of assessing plain film lumbar spine radiographs for the presence of developmental canal stenosis would be to first consider four easily visualised and relatively independent features on the AP projection: the interpedicular distance; the visibility of the posterior intervertebral joints; the height of posterior intervertebral joint; the interlaminar space width. Secondly, examination of three features on the lateral projection film may help to confirm these abnormalities: Eisenstein's measure which largely correlates with interpedicular distance; pedicle length largely correlating with interlaminar space width; pedicle thickness at L5 largely correlating with the posterior intervertebral joint height and often not easy to visualise. In addition the fact that men tend to have slightly narrower canals than women should be considered.

Despite the significant relationships of plain film features with canal size, the application of predictive techniques of this kind to the clinical management of patients is limited. In many instances clinical features will determine treatment or prognosis regardless of plain film measurements. Furthermore, myelography, CT or MRI scanning which provide so much more information than plain film radiology will be performed in many patients whatever the latter may show.

The observation that cervical developmental stenosis is part of a generalised skeletal misproportion provides a new insight into the pathogenesis of developmental stenosis. Although these observations are statistically significant, only 22% of the variation in developmental canal size can be related to somatotype. The factors responsible for the remaining variation of canal size may include other aspects of somatotype, that cannot be adequately assessed by standard anthropometry, as well as inherited or acquired sources of variation unique to individual subjects. Inaccuracy in the measurement of the cervical radiographs or anthropometric variables is unlikely to be responsible for much of the residual variation as the standard errors of these measurements are small particularly when compared to the total range of each of these variables (Nightingale, 1986).

Although the large standard error of the estimate prevents accurate prediction of cervical canal size from somatotype, the presence of a relatively short upper arm and a long trunk in a patient with spinal symptoms may alert the physician or surgeon to the possibility of developmental cervical canal stenosis and consequently the greater risk of the expression of degenerative spine disease.

References

Babin, E. (1980), Radiology of the narrow lumbar canal. In: *The narrow lumbar canal. Radiologic signs and surgery*, eds. A. Wackenheim & E. Babin, pp. 1–10. Springer-Verlag, New York.

Cameron, N. (1978), The methods of auxological anthropometry. In: *Human Growth*, eds. F. Falkener & J. M. Tanner, pp. 35–90. Plenum Press, New York.

Eisenstein, S. (1976), Measurement of the lumbar spinal canal in two racial groups, *Clinical Orthopaedics and Related Research*, **115**, 42–6.

Eisenstein, S. (1977), The morphometry and pathological anatomy of the lumbar spine in South African negroes and Caucasoids with specific reference to spinal stenosis, *Journal of Bone and Joint Surgery*, **59B**, 173–80.

Epstein, B. S., Epstein, J. A. & Jones, M.D. (1977), Cervical spinal stenosis, *Radiologic Clinics of North America*, **15**, 215–25.

Hinck, V. S. & Sachdev, N. S. (1966), Developmental stenosis of the cervical spinal canal, *Brain*, **89**, 27–36.

Kim, J. O. (1983), Factor analysis. In: *SPSS Users Guide*, eds. N. H. Nie, C. H. Hull & J. G. Jenkins, pp. 468–514. McGraw, New York.

Lawrence, J. S., de Graaf, R. & Laine, V. A. I. (1963), Degeneration of joint disease in random samples and occupational groups. In: *Epidemiology of Chronic Rheumatism*, eds. J. H. Kellgren, M. R. Jeffrey & J. Ball, p. 98. Blackwell Scientific, Oxford.

Lutter, L. D. (1978), Achondroplasia – clinical manifestations and neurological significance. In: *Spinal deformities and neurological dysfunction*, eds. S. N. Chou, & E. L. Seljeskog. Raven, New York.

McRae, D.L. (1977), Radiology of the lumbar spinal canal. In: *Lumbar spondylosis: diagnosis, management and surgical treatment*, eds. P. R. Weinstein, G. Ehni & C. B. Wilson, pp. 92–114. Year Book of Medicine, London.

Nie, N. H., Hull, C. H. & Jenkins, J. G. (1983), *SPSS Users Guide*, McGraw, New York.

Nightingale, S. (1986), Developmental vertebral canal stenosis. A clinical, radiological, anthropometric and genetic study, MD Thesis, University of London.

Nurick, S. (1972), The pathogenesis of the spinal cord disorder associated with cervical spondylosis, *Brain*, **95**, 87–100.

Payne, E. E. & Spillane, J. D. (1957), The cervical spine: an anatomico-pathological study of 70 specimens (using a special technique) with particular reference to the problem of cervical spondylosis, *Brain*, **80**, 571–93.

Postacchini, F., Ripani, M. & Carpano, S. (1983). Morphometry of the lumbar vertebrae. An anatomic study of two Causcasoid ethnic groups, *Clinical Orthopaedics and Related Research*, **172**, 296–303.

Roberts, G. M. (1978), Lumbar stenosis, MD Thesis, University of London.

Verbiest, H. (1975), Pathomorphologic aspects of developmental lumbar stenosis, *Orthopedic Clinics of North America*, **6**, 177–96.

Verbiest, H. (1976), *Neurogenic intermittent claudication. With special reference to stenosis of the lumbar vertebral canal*, Elsevier, New York.

Verbiest, H. (1980), Stenosis of the bony lumbar vertebral canal. In: *The narrow lumbar canal. Radiologic signs and surgery*. Eds A. Wackenheim & E. Babin, pp. 115–46. Springer-Verlag, New York.

Weinstein, P.R. (1980), The application of anatomy and pathophysiology in the management of lumbar spine disease, *Clinical Neurosurgery*, **27**, 517–40.

Discussion

Fairbank: Of the 100 patients you looked at, how many of them actually had a relatively narrow cervical canal? If one has a small number of patients at that end of the spectrum, does that not put you in difficulties about drawing these conclusions? I appreciate that statistics must take that into account.

Nightingale (in reply): The answers you get depend on the questions you ask. I considered canal size to be a continuous variable with a normal distribution. In the population that I studied, this is what I found, and therefore the appropriate statistic was multiple regression analysis in which the dependent variable has to be normally distributed. Now, an alternative would have been to go out and find grossly atypical people who have very narrow canals, for example, people with achondroplasia, and compare them to a normal group. In that situation, we are looking at a dichotomous dependent variable and one would have to use a quite different technique such as discriminant analyses. I have measured a lot of spines of patients with achondroplasia, and there are some features in common with those with idiopathic stenosis, but there are also many features which are different. For example, in the achondroplastic, the size of the lumbar-spine canal does not increase from L1 to L5, in contrast to a normal population where it does increase.

Eisenstein: I would like to congratulate Dr Nightingale. I had got bored with the subject of spinal stenosis, but I think that this work has elevated the subject onto a whole new plane by bringing in the somatotypes. I am fascinated by it.

Nelson: I was interested in your talk where you mentioned achondroplasia, because, as you know, the achondroplastic has got short proximal segments and a relatively long trunk. It does seem to me that occasionally you see people who have achondroplasia-like features without the full expression of the condition. Perhaps this is associated with a genetic basis for spinal stenosis. May I share Mr Eisenstein's congratulations to you for this fascinating work.

Nightingale (in reply): Some families have been reported with an autosomal dominant disorder similar to achondroplasia but with much milder features. These 'hypochondrioplastics' would certainly be worth studying.

Nelson: I wondered at one stage if we were seeing some form of rickets in patients with spinal stenosis. Because in rickets, as you know, you get a shortening of long bones through disturbance of the growth plate. The growth of the AP diameter of the spinal canal is dependant on the inclusion of part of the posterior elements with the centrum. There is a growth plate between the two primary centres near the centre of one side of the posterior arc of the centrum. If you had some disturbance of that growth plate early on in life, you might end up with a narrow canal.

Nightingale: At what age does rickets affect the development in that way?

Nelson: We know for example that there were a large number of children who developed bow legs which corrected spontaneously, they bowed soon after birth and they seemed to improve and at the time there was some talk about whether or not this could represent some form of temporary vitamin D deficiency. I just wondered again whether early on in life this could be a factor.

Nightingale (in reply): It may well be.

Fairbank: Is spinal stenosis related to social class? Social class was obviously one of the potential factors of rickets when this condition was more common in this country?

Nightingale (in reply): Well certainly there is a social class distinction in height. Tall people become upwardly mobile and short people are down there somewhere! I do not know about shape, that is another matter!

Corlett: When you showed your early distribution you described it as a normal distribution, but it looked rather skewed to me. It did occur to me that the other dimensions that you have taken have a similar shape and that you might reduce the errors by introducing some correction?

Nightingale (in reply): Yes, it did not look perfectly bell-shaped but there are standard statistical techniques for checking whether ones data conform to a normal distribution and the probability that it is, or is not, part of a normal distribution. I used analysis of probability plots to show that the dependent variables were normally distributed.

Multivariate analysis – an application in rheumatology

10.1 Introduction

Multivariate analysis provides a powerful statistical methodology for considering the inter-relationships between several 'independent' variables (e.g. age, weight loss, mood) and a 'dependent' variable (e.g. backache). It recognises that the independent variables may themselves interact, so that simply defining the link between each one and the dependent variable (i.e. univariate analysis) provides an oversimplified assessment of the way in which the data are related. It might reveal, for example, that weight loss related to depression accounts for all the weight change related to backache in a particular group of patients.

There are a variety of techniques available in multivariate analysis (Armitage, 1971). In some, the way in which independent variables can be combined to discriminate between different values of the dependent variable is explored (discriminant function analysis). Other techniques group variables which appear to relate closely to each other (factor analysis), or group cases which have similar values for particular sets of variables (cluster analysis). Multiple regression analysis calculates the relative strength of the links between each independent variable and the dependent variable. All these techniques have similar strengths, weaknesses and pitfalls. This chapter uses examples from rheumatology to illustrate some of them.

10.2 Application in rheumatology

When rheumatologists assess the severity of rheumatoid arthritis (RA) they use a variety of clinical and laboratory data to do so. Using multiple regression analysis we have calculated the relative contribution of each individual 'cue' to the decision-making policy of individual doctors (Kirwan *et al.*, 1983b, 1984). Each was asked to score the degree of change in RA in patients for whom ten clinical cues were known before and after a course of treatment. The regression analysis used (Frane, 1981) was designed to limit the number of variables in the regression equation to about six (see below) and the ability of the equation to match the actual judgments made by the doctors was gauged from the square of the correlation between them and the calculated values produced from the equation (R^2 – the square of the multiple correlation coefficient). R^2 for many of these equations was very high (>0.75), leading us to conclude that they were acceptable models of the doctors' policy for making these clinical judgements. This technique has been called 'policy capturing' (Hammond *et al.*, 1975) or 'clinical judgment analysis' (Kirwan *et al.*, 1983b).

The relative contribution of each variable to a policy model is best measured as its relative contribution to R^2 (Hoffman, 1960) and can be illustrated using a bar chart. In the example given (Figure 10.1), six variables make major contributions to the judgment policy of doctor J. Using this form of multivariate analysis has resulted in many insights into rheumatologists' decision-making, which are reviewed more fully elsewhere (Chaput de Saintonge *et al.*, 1989). Four of the more important conditions are that:

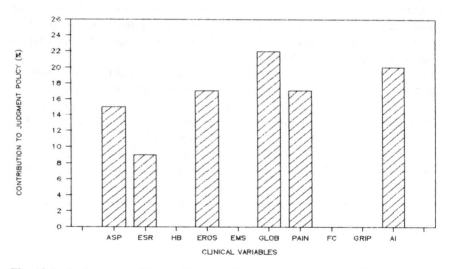

Fig. 10.1   Judgement policy for Doctor J. Relative importance of clinical variables is represented by the height of the bars: ASP = aspirin consumption; ESR = erythrocyte sedimentation rate; HB = haemoglobin; EROS = erosions; EMS = early morning stiffness; GLOB = patient's overall assessment, PAIN = pain score; FC = functional capacity; GRIP = grip strength; AI = articular index

(1) rheumatologists in three continents adopt a wide variety of different policies (Kirwan *et al.*, 1983a, 1984, 1985);

(2) each maintains a stable policy over long periods (Kirwan & Currey, 1984);

(3) physicians are not able accurately to describe their judgement policies (Kirwan *et al.*, 1986); but

(4) they can modify their policies when provided with the detailed information revealed by the policy models (Kirwan *et al.*, 1983c, 1988).

These findings illustrate the strength of this form of multivariate analysis. Other tests have been performed which explore the weaknesses of the technique, so that they might be avoided during these practical applications.

10.3 Illustrations of weaknesses in multivariate techniques

The results of multivariate analysis may be particularly sensitive to idiosyncrasies in the data on which the analysis is based. The equations in Table 10.1 illustrate two policy models calculated from the same set of patient data except that values from a particular patient were omitted from the second calculation. There are clear differences between the results obtained. In general, such instability in the calculated results may follow from the inclusion of 'outlier' patients who are not truly part of the patient population under study, or from the availability of too few cases compared to the number of variables included in the equation. There should be at least five cases for every variable in the equation and some authors recommend as many as 15 (Dawes & Corrigan, 1974).

Multiple regression analysis may include all the available variables in the equation and in doing so will obtain the maximum value for R^2. In practice such equations will lack biological credibility. For example, it is not possible to consider more than seven variables at once during decision making (Miller, 1956). Removal of a few variables usually makes little difference to R^2, and a balance must be sought between R^2 and the number of variables included (Figure 10.2). Two common approaches to elimina-

Table 10.1 Judgement policy equations for doctor M35

(A)	When 50 cases are included: Judgement = 2.8 − 61 × erosions − 18 × functional capacity
(B)	When 49 cases are included: Judgement = 2.4 − 56 × crosions − 14 × functional capacity

J. Kirwan

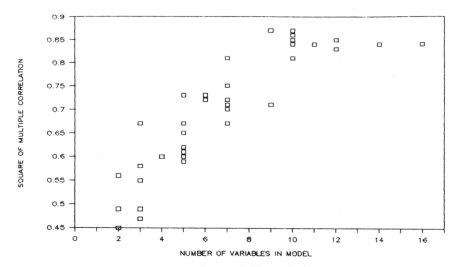

Fig. 10.2 R^2 *vs* number of variables for judgement policy models Policy models from four doctors were recalculated nine times each with different 'penalties' for including variables (see text). The number of variables in each recalculated model is shown in relation to R^2, the ability of the model to fit the doctors' judgements

ting variables may unfortunately produce very different results. In the first, variables are sequentially included in the equation because they make significant contribution to R^2, given those variables already included. The alternative method starts by including all the variables, then dropping

Table 10.2 Model robustness in 80% subsamples of patients

Doctor code	Number of variables in model	Number of variables in model included in at least four 80% models[a]	Number of variables not in model but included in more than one 80% model[a]
MO4	5	5	0
M29	7	4[b]	1[d]
M36	5	5	4[e]
M43	5	5	0
PO4	4	3[c]	0
Total	22	26	5

[a] 80% models are those calculated using random 80% subsets of the cases
[b] The relative contributions to R^2 for the omitted variables were 10%, 7%, 6%
[c] The relative contribution to R^2 for the omitted variable was 6%
[d] Included in three 80% models
[e] Included in two 80% models each

in turn those which make the least significant contribution to R^2, until a predetermined limit is reached. We have adopted a third technique – all subsets regression analysis (Frane, 1981), which reviews all combinations of the variables and chooses that which gives the highest R^2 when balanced against a 'penalty' for including larger numbers of variables. Table 10.2 shows that the equations which result from this approach are relatively insensitive to large changes in the data while still providing high values for R^2. Table 10.2 was derived by recalculating models from five randomly chosen rheumatologists five times each, using only 80% of the cases each time (randomly selected) (Kirwan, 1983). The number of occasions on which variables were included in these five recalculated models was compared to their inclusion in the initial model based on all the cases. The results show that the majority of variables included in the original model appear in most of the recalculated models (22/26, 85%) and few of those omitted appear in more than one recalculated model (5/74, 7%).

10.4 Cluster analysis

Clinical judgement policy models were obtained for a random sample of 48 UK rheumatologists in the United Kingdom (Kirwan *et al.*, 1984). A second multivariate technique, cluster analysis (Dixon *et al.*, 1981), was then used to discover if the doctors could be classified into naturally occurring groups and if these groups had differing policies. Identification of clusters is based on a partially subjective interpretation of the results of the analysis, which may itself be performed in a variety of ways analagous to those of multiple regression analysis. We identified five clusters of doctors based on various demographic features (Table 10.3). The remaining seven

Table 10.3 Cluster analysis of respondents based on demographic data

Cluster name	Number in cluster	Published papers	Type of appointment[a]	Geography[b]	City[c]	Age
D1	3	None	DGH1	–	–	older
D2	12	Few	DGH2	Midlands & SE England	–	younger
D3	4	Some	T	SE England	–	older
D4	13	Few	A	SE England	+	middle
D5	10	Few	T	–	+	younger

[a] DGHI = District General Hospital with only one rheumatologist;
 DGH2 = District General Hospital with more than one rheumatologist;
 T = Teaching Hospital; A = Academic
[b] – = no specific geography defined
[c] + = large city; – = not a large city

Table 10.4   Summary of cluster variables

Cluster	Four major variables		
D2	GRIP, ESR, EMS, GLOBAL		
D4	GRIP, ESR, EMS,	AI	
D5	GRIP, ESR		AI, ASP

For key to variables see Figure 10.1

rheumatologists did not fall into any groups. The major clinical variables in the combined policy models of the main clusters are shown in Table 10.3. Although this was not a powerful analysis, it does seem to have identified differences in the judgement models of different types of rheumatologist.

10.5 Conclusion

Multivariate techniques are powerful tools for data analysis which can be readily applied by computers. Unlike simple statistical tests, there are many different ways of performing each analysis and results will differ depending on the method chosen. In addition, results may be sensitive to idiosyncrasies in the data set or the inclusion of too few cases. Even with a given approach, interpretation of the analysis may be subjective. There are no statistical tests by which to gauge the likelihood of a misleading result. In these circumstances precautions must be taken to maximise the stability of the results of analysis, their biological credibility, and their applicability in new data sets. Within these limitations the use of multivariate analysis has been productive and will continue to be so.

References

Armitage, P. (1971), *Statistical Methods in Medical Research*, Blackwell Scientific Publications, London.

Chaput de Saintonge, D. M., Fisch, H. U., Joyce, C. R. B. & Kirwan, J. R. (1989), Clinical judgement: why and how to improve it. In: *Human Psychopharmacology: Measures and Methods 2*, eds. Hindmarch & Stonier, pp. 271–7. John Wiley & Sons Ltd., London.

Dawes, R. M. & Corrigan, B. (1974), Linear models in decision making, *Psychological Bulletin*, **81**, 95–106.

Dixon, W. J., Brown, M. B. & Engelman, L. (eds.) (1981), *Biochemical computer programs, P-series*, University of California Press, Berkeley.

Frane, J. W. (1981), All possible subsets regression. In: *Biochemical computer programs, P-series*, eds. W. J. Dixon, M. B. Brown & L. Engleman. University of California Press, Berkeley.

Hammond, K. R., Stewart, T. R., Brehmner, B. & Steinmann, D. O. (1975), Social judgement theory. In: *Human Judgment and Decision Making*, eds. M. F.

Kaplan, & S. Schwartz. Academic Press, New York.

Hoffman, P. J., (1960), The paramorphic representation of clinical judgement, *Psychological Bulletin*, **57**, 116–31.

Kirwan, J. R. (1983), Social judgement theory and rheumatic diseases: application of clinical judgement analysis to rheumatoid arthritis, MD Thesis, University of London.

Kirwan, J. R., Barnes, C. G., Davies, P. G. & Currey, H. L. F. (1988), Analysis of clinical judgement helps to improve agreement in the assessment of rheumatoid arthritis, *Annals of the Rheumatic Diseases*, **47**, 138–43.

Kirwan, J. R., Bellamy, N., Condon, H., Buchanan, W. W. & Barnes, C. G. (1983a), Judgement of 'current disease activity' in rheumatoid arthritis – an international comparison, *Journal of Rheumatology*, **10**, 901–5.

Kirwan, J. R., Brooks, P. M. & Currey, H. L. F. (1985), Measuring physicians' judgement – the use of clinical data by Australian rheumatologists, *Australia and New Zealand Journal of Medicine*, **15**, 738–44.

Kirwan, J. R., Chaput de Saintonge, D. M., Joyce, C. R. B. & Currey, H. L. F. (1983b), Clinical judgement in rheumatoid arthritis II. Judging 'current disease activity' in rheumatoid arthritis, *Annals of the Rheumatic Diseases*, **42**, 648–51.

Kirwan, J. R., Chaput de Saintonge, D. M., Joyce, C. R. B. & Currey, H. L. F. (1983c), Advances in assessing rheumatoid arthritis – a review of the symposium/workshop, *British Journal of Rheumatology*, (suppl.), 95–7.

Kirwan, J. R., Chaput de Saintonge, D. M., Joyce, C. R. B. & Currey, H. L. F. (1984), Clinical judgement in rheumatoid arthritis III. British rheumatologists' judgements of 'change in response to therapy', *Annals of the Rheumatic Diseases*, **43**, 695–97.

Kirwan, J. R., Chaput de Saintonge, D. M., Joyce, C. R. B., Holmes, J. & Currey, H. L. F. (1986), Inability of rheumatolologists to describe their true policies for assessing rheumatoid arthritis, *Annals of the Rheumatic Diseases*, **45**, 156–61.

Kirwan, J. R. & Currey, H. L. F. (1984), Clinical judgement in rheumatoid arthritis IV. Rheumatologists' judgements are stable over long periods, *Annals of the Rheumatic Diseases*, **43**, 695–97.

Miller, G. A. (1956), The magical number seven, plus or minus two: some limits on our capacity for processing information, *Psychological Review*, **63**, 81–97.

Discussion

Jayson: As one of the chaps that filled in your form, you seem to assume that the doctor uses the same judgement policy throughout a variety of judgement tasks. Is that a fair assumption?

Kirwan (in reply): No it is not. We have worked in an extremely well-defined area which we chose in advance (using our own judgement). All the mathematical ways of combining data are likely to be in strictly limited areas. Nobody is going to be able to replace you for deciding that this is a patient who has to be treated with penicillamine and you have to decide whether or not they have got better.

We have done some work that has shown that over long periods of time, within that small catchment area, doctors use the same judgement policies. When we did the analysis a year later, which is the longest that has ever been done, these doctors were operating very close to the same policy that they had been using the year before. We are currently going through a batch of half a dozen people who we have analysed 5 years later and I will let you know the results in due course.

Rowland: We had one speaker this morning who came from the same city as you (Matthew) who has warned us against using computer techniques that rely on assuming independence of variables when making decision judgements. Can you, in fact, use multiple regression techniques on variables which are clearly correlated with one another?

Kirwan (in reply): This is a good point and is the reason why I said that you have to take precautions against it. We did this by using the all subsets analysis, by double checking data sets, by repeating over many times and by limiting the extent to which we were prepared to draw conclusions from the data and drawing only simple conclusions from it. If you take these precautions, then yes you can use this technique. Our analysis works on the basis of recognising that the data are inter-correlated. That is the whole point about it, so in fact I agree with the previous speakers. The way we are using it in this analysis is recognising the problem and using that to help us to build sensible models.

Main: I was interested in your presentation. We have been using multiple regression models for about 10 years on back pain patients, trying to disentangle different things, and I have a couple of observations which I think might be relevant to you. The first is that these techniques have been applied over quite a wide range, within the field of back pain, to investigations trying to disentangle the relevant information. I think it is quite important before people adopt it uncritically to remember that what you are testing with each regression equation is a particular model. I have been to one or two conferences where people have come along triumphant with their computer printout with the most amazing findings, with the justification that because the computer produced it, it must be right. At a meeting I was at some years ago, a Dutch physician produced his multiple regression model and found that the single most important influence in patients with back pain was irritation of the foot! What had happened was that there had been a completely accidental finding and he had not taken the steps that you have suggested to cross-validate his findings. I think it is important not to place too much reliance on the actual number crunching itself, you have got to have some questions that can be formally defined, as you have done, in the first instance.

Kirwan: I would like to reinforce your point. He might have come back and said that it was related to pain in the sacro-iliac joint. He might have made exactly the same modelling mistake, but you would not have picked it up because it did not have obvious biological inaccuracy. You must not take results simply at face value and it is as difficult an area as laboratory technique for measuring rheumatoid factor or whatever, and when people stand up and present their results, they must explain exactly how they were obtained. They must have expert help. I have worked with experts in this area who do all the hard work for me and you cannot get away from that.

Whither classification of back pain syndromes?

Attempting to classify back pain syndromes is like looking into a muddy
fish pond in the hope of recognising some of the species lurking in the
depths of the pool. We see one or two recognisable varieties but know that
there are many as yet unrecognised specimens hiding in the murky water.
There has been some progress in recent years in the classification of
syndromes producing root pain. We are fairly clear about root pain from a
disc protrusion when the outer annulus is intact, or from an extrusion or
sequestration when there has been a complete fissure of the annulus with
nuclear disruption. We understand how the disc material compromises the
space in the central or root canal affecting the nerve root producing
symptoms and signs in the legs. Some of the pathophysiology of nerve
function has still to be resolved but the syndrome is recognisable from the
history and examination, investigations confirm the causative pathology
and expeditious and appropriate surgical treatment will give a good result.

We also have little problem with the syndrome of root entrapment from
degenerative changes causing lateral canal stenosis. The pathology may be
bony degeneration from a posterior vertebral bar, or a thickened lamina or
osteophytes adjacent to the apophyseal joint; there may be thickened soft
tissue from disc degeneration, capsular thickening of the apophyseal joint,
synovial swelling or soft tissue related to a pars defect. Not infrequently
there is a dynamic component related to abnormal intersegmental
vertebral movement. This degenerative pathology produces pain in a root
distribution. We still need to know more about the distinctive quality of
this root pain when compared with root pain from a disc protrusion, and
we still do not know why straight leg raising is generally unimpaired with
this type of pathology, but the syndrome is clear.

Central spinal stenosis producing the symptoms of neurogenic claudication is also a recognisable syndrome, but the pathophysiological mechan-

ism has not been fully explained. We do not understand why one patient has a complete occlusion and another with the same symptoms has only partial encroachment; why many patients have multiple level lesions, why a central stenosis may produce symptoms only in one leg, and why peripheral vascular disease often coexists.

The syndrome of root claudication is distinct from root entrapment from lateral stenosis but may be the remaining symptom after a classical root entrapment has resolved. Why root claudication can occur after a disc protrusion, or after root entrapment with stenosis of the root canal, or with a complete central canal occlusion, is not understood. The syndromes merge but are becoming less confused.

Back pain syndromes which produce symptoms and signs of nerve root involvement with pain in the leg are fairly well recognisable and there is much general agreement. It is in the area of back pain alone, or back and referred pain, that confusion exists. In fact, there is so much difficulty that some advocate a departure from the traditional hierarchial classification.

From antiquity there have been different philosophies in medicine and this is still characteristic of our approach to the classification of back pain syndromes. Hippocrates, who died in 377 BC, founded a School of Medicine on the Island of Cos. Its philosophy could be summarised as a study of the diseased, considering the total sick man. There was a contrasting School of Medicine in Knidos which emphasised the disease, focusing on symptoms and pathology. Western medicine has attempted to identify the pain source from a study of the symptoms and signs, and although diagnosis of the pain source can be difficult, particularly in the area of back pain, we have no licence to adopt an alternative approach.

The patient attempts to describe their pain experience and we apply detective skills to identify the pain source. In the area of back pain the difficulties are so great that we are tempted to adopt a different approach, but in spite of these difficulties, the hierarchial classification of symptomatic pathology has stood the test of time and should not be abandoned. What are the problems? They arise in part from patients but also from the physician.

The problem with the patient is that we, the doctors, cannot rely on being told the truth; the patient may be consciously deceiving us for some gainful purpose. Alternatively they deceive themselves, with a pain experience which does not match up to a pain source in the lumbar spine. As yet, we are not able to estimate the size of this non-organic problem, but it undoubtedly exists.

Even when a patient presents an understandable account of pain experience and this does match up to abnormal objective signs, we are not skilled at relating symptoms and signs to the responsible pathology in the spine. Our clinical skills have not reached the stage where we can confidently identify the source of pain when the symptoms are in the back alone.

Sophisticated investigations reveal all manner of pathology in the spine; this may be symptomless. Conversely we suspect that many a pain source is not necessarily associated with demonstrable pathology. This is the dilemma with the patient.

The problem with the physician is both semantics and tradition. The International Society for the Study of the Lumbar Spine attempted to resolve the problem of language by introducing a Glossary of Spinal Terminology in 1984. Although this has been accepted by its members, there is no compulsion for physicians in other spine societies to use the same terminology. Physicians are using different language to describe identical symptoms, signs and conditions.

Our interest in the lumbar spine has evolved from many different traditions. The surgeon has been taught his trade from previous generations of barber surgeons. The rheumatologist has grown from another branch of the tree, whilst chiropractors and osteopaths look further into history for their origins. Our basic scientists have followed another path. It is not surprising that when we meet together to discuss classification of back pain syndromes, we are like a multilingual society trying to communicate without translators. How can we hope to identify and classify back pain syndromes when we understand neither our patients nor each other?

We recognise that our objective in understanding back pain is to identify the patient's pain source and so develop a classification. There can be several approaches to this quest. First, the clinician can attempt to identify syndrome A and syndrome B with defined criteria, and then look for significant differences in observed pathology in the two syndromes, or differences in response to treatment of the two syndromes. If there are significant differences he may be justified in concluding that these two syndromes have a different pain source and go so far as to suggest pathology which is responsible. He may then break down these syndromes into sub-groups and assess them again to extend his classification.

An approach is to recognise pathology A and pathology B by some investigation, and compare symptoms and signs in patients who exhibit these two pathologies and also compare response to treatment. Significant differences would suggest that these pathologies are related to a pain source. There are unfortunately few such comparative studies.

The chapters in this book, however, do suggest how we might divide our patients into groups in the area of pain patterns, abnormal signs, or response to treatment. Unfortunately, most of us talk about some syndrome that we think we can recognise by certain criteria, and we treat such patients with a particular therapy we believe will help. The criteria of diagnosis and the methods of treatment are rarely defined and we are slow to compare and analyse our results. Chapters in this book about repeatability of measurement and differences of interpretation, illustrate the difficulties of comparing results between examiners. It is not surprising that progress is slow.

Some may ask whether our quest for a pain source and a hierarchial classification is justified. At this moment in time, are we not better advised to cluster patients by specific types of pain or by their response to treatment? Without identifying the pain source however, our symptomatic cluster will probably be too large. We need to focus on the pathology responsible for the pain source in order to know the natural history of this particular conditon. Without understanding its natural course how can we hope to modify it? Similarly, if we do not understand the pathology responsible for the condition, we shall be ignorant of its aetiology and helpless to prevent it in the next generation. A scientific approach to back pain demands proper classification.

So what are the hopes for the future? Whither classification? First, for the clinician there is scope for improved observation. There are signs, as yet undiscovered, to be recognised and described. There are signs which will change diurnally and with physical activity and we need to understand their significance. There is opportunity for identifying those symptoms and signs which can be grouped together and weighted to identify back pain syndromes. For example, the extension catch is a common sign which we do not understand; it has not even been analysed in biomechanical terms. There are many similar signs and symptoms whose relevance are at the present time lost. We are beginning to quantify abnormal signs, such as range of movement, and better understand examination error. Computer analysis should also help us to understand the diagnostic significance of our observations.

Secondly, we may expect progress in the area of pain behaviour. In order to classify back pain syndromes we have to unravel the complexity of inappropriate behaviours. How much can we rely on the history given? How many of the abnormal signs we detect are compatible with the spinal pathology? How many are distorted by subjectivity and patients' distress?

Finally, although we may believe that the new sophisticated investigations will help in diagnosis, this is but the beginning of useful investigative procedures. Pathology does not mean pain, but with time we should have procedures which identify the pain source.

The pond is murky with only a few recognisable species, but there are signs that the water will clear and that one day we shall have a satisfactory back pain classification.

An analysis of the histories of patients with common syndromes of back pain from a computer database

12.1 Introduction

Physicians with an interest in low back pain are aware that that there is a spectrum of clinical presentations in their patients with backache. A number of diagnostic schemes for the classification of back pain syndromes have been published, but it is rare for the author to give a sufficiently precise description for these classifications to be in general use. Even when a precise definition of the syndrome is given, it is difficult for clinicians to give an exact description and the weight of the various criteria used. At this hospital we have developed a computerised back pain interview system (Pynsent & Fairbank, 1989) capable of obtaining a detailed history from patients with back pain. A validation study of its reliability compared to a standard clinical interview has been performed (Thomas *et al.*, 1989), and this confirms a high level of agreement between clinician and computer interview. The object of this chapter is to use the database of the Birmingham Back Pain Interview to define the history criteria of patients classified by an experienced clinician into five clinical groups, using all the data available to him.

12.2 Materials and methods

The Birmingham Back Pain Interview system consists of a microcomputer-based software package and light-pen patient interface for the patient. After a brief introduction, patients are left unattended seated in front of the computer screen. They are presented with a series of questions that are either single choice, multiple choice, or graphics, such as homunculi (for pain patterns) or thermometers (for linear analogue pain scales). The duration of the interview is between 30 and 60 min. There is a total of 253 screens of questions but most patients are only exposed to about

180 screens. This is because of branching logic within the programme that makes the presentation of some questions dependent on previous responses.

For this study, one author (JCTF) retrospectively reviewed 312 patients referred to his clinic. He classified each of them into one of five groups. All the patients had been seen and examined by him and were investigated and treated according to current practice. The classification was made on the basis of all the clinical, radiological, biochemical and haematogical data available, as well as the response to physiotherapy and other conservative therapy, and surgery where it was indicated. The classification is based on a group of syndromes suggested by Fairbank & Hall (1990). The groups and their perceived pathologies are:

Type 1. Facet syndrome

Type 2. Discogenic

Type 3. Combined disc pathology and root compression

Type 4. Neurogenic claudication

Type 5. Unclassifiable.

Patients were classified into these groups from the case notes, results of investigations, and response to treatment. The classification was performed 3–18 months after the initial consultation.

Three types of data were available from the database, namely: continuous, single choice categorical, and multiple choice categorical. The continuous data were analysed by a one-way analysis of variance and the categorical data were investigated in the following manner. First a chi-squared test was used to compare the five group classification with the response to each question. This identified those questions that produced a statistically significant variation from the result if the answering had been random ($p < 0.05$). It was assumed that these questions were responsible for most of the clinical difference between the groups. The contingency table frequencies for these questions were then used to calculate likelihood ratios and their natural logarithms.

A likelihood ratio is the ratio of the proportion of cases with an attribute in the group in question to the proportion of cases with that attribute who are not in the group. Thus if 70% of patients with diagnosis A were men and 35% of patients with diagnosis B were men, the likelihood ratio would be calculated by dividing 70 by 35 to obtain 2.0. This means that a patient who has diagnosis A is twice as likely to be a man than a patient who has diagnosis B. It also means that if a diseased patient is a man, he is more likely to be suffering from diagnosis A than B.

This technique has been used by Macartney (1977) and Knill-Jones

(1987) who have equated likelihood ratios and their logarithms with the term 'weight of evidence' for a particular diagnosis. A likelihood ratio above 1.0 is considered evidence in favour of a particular diagnosis and a ratio less than 1.0 is considered evidence against a particular diagnosis. It can be shown that Bayes's theorem for calculating posterior probability can be rewritten as:

$$\text{posterior odds} = \text{prior odds} \times \text{likelihood ratio}$$

where prior odds are the ratio between the probability of a diagnosis and the probability of its compliment. The posterior odds are the new odds after the observation of a new attribute. Using this theorem the posterior odds are progressively refined with each new observation which imparts its own 'weight of evidence'. Starting with the initial prior odds, the final posterior odds, after observing all the 'clues', are obtained by a series of multiplications of the likelihood ratios. This can be made easier and more intuitive by taking the natural logarithm of the likelihood ratios. This is because logarithms can be added rather than multiplied to produce the desired result. The logarithms of the likelihood ratios now produce a score that has the property of being positive, if the evidence is in favour of a particular diagnosis, and negative if the evidence is against the diagnosis. If the weights of evidence of an observed symptom is added to the logarithm of the prior odds of each diagnosis, the diagnosis with the largest score is the most likely diagnosis. This is only true if the assumption of independence of all symptoms is made. This assumption is impossible to prove or disprove. However, considering the nature of the questions in our back pain interview system it seems likely that this assumption is false. Whilst this limits the suitability of this approach as a diagnostic procedure, the weights of evidence indicate the degree to which a question is important in describing the groups.

12.3 Results

The continuous variables of age, height, weight, and standing height/sitting height ratio, were analysed by one-way analysis of variance. The only feature found to have a statistically significant distribution was age ($p < 0.001$). The mean ages of the groups are shown in Table 12.1. It can be seen that on average patients with type 1 are younger and patients with type 4 pain are older.

Table 12.2 shows the frequencies of each of the five groups in the sample. Analysis of 34 single choice questions produced 34 contingency tables. Analysis of 24 multiple choice questions produced 211 contingency tables (as each n choice question was split into n tables). Chi squared analysis of all 245 tables showed 26 tables with a probability value of less

Table 12.1 Average age for five group classification of 312 cases of back pain. Significant difference ($p < 0.001$) by analysis of variance.

Description	Type	Mean age
Facet syndrome	1	38.5
Discogenic	2	43.0
Discogenic and root compression	3	41.0
Neurogenic claudication	4	61.7
Unclassifiable	5	45.5

Table 12.2 Frequency table for a five group classification of back pain applied to 312 cases

Description	Type	Frequency	%
Facet syndrome	1	64	20.51
Discogenic	2	129	41.35
Discogenic and root compression	3	21	6.73
Neurogenic claudication	4	39	12.50
Unclassifiable	5	59	18.91
Total		312	100.00

than 0.05. As each table consisted of at least a present–absent state for an attribute, a minimum of two sets of five weights of evidence was produced for each table (each set corresponding to the weights of evidence for when the attribute was present and absent). A total of 55 sets of weights were produced. The questions and their weights of evidence (logarithm of likelihood ratios) are shown in Table 12.3. Tables 12.4–12.8 show the questions ordered by weights for each of the five groups and show the features of each of the groups in order of importance. Table 12.9 shows an ordered list of the 'best questions' to ask in order to discriminate the groups. This was obtained by ordering the questions by the range of the weights for the five groups. This is because the question with the largest difference between the maximum and minimum weight will clearly be the most discriminating. The most discriminating feature was answering 'No' to the question, 'Is the reason for you coming here back pain?'. It should be remembered that the patients answering were all referred with symptoms associated with spinal disease, this latter response would indicate another site of pain (perhaps the thighs or legs).

12.4 Conclusions and discussion

While there is a certain tautology inherent in analysing the clinical features of syndromes that have been classified largely on clinical grounds, the

Table 12.3 Weights of evidence for five group classification of back pain. The positive weights indicate support for the diagnosis, negative weights indicate evidence against the diagnosis

Question	1	2	Type 3	4	5
Is the reason for you coming here back pain — no	0.00	-1.86	2.18	1.21	0.02
Is the reason for you coming here back pain — yes	0.04	0.04	-0.19	-0.07	0.00
Is the reason for you coming here arm or hand pain — yes	-1.03	-0.48	-0.97	0.45	1.07
Is the reason for you coming here arm or hand pain — no	0.10	0.06	0.09	-0.07	-0.20
Is the reason for you coming here leg pain — yes	-1.00	-0.25	0.67	0.53	0.31
Is the reason for you coming here leg pain — no	0.55	0.21	-1.37	-0.76	-0.33
Is your present pain worst in your back — yes	-0.20	0.66	-2.04	-0.52	0.04
Is your present pain worst in your legs or feet — yes	0.41	-1.03	1.10	0.34	-0.31
Is your present pain the same severity in your legs and back — no	0.00	0.10	0.00	0.58	0.39
Is your pain continuous — yes	-1.01	0.29	-0.85	0.05	0.46
Is your pain intermittent — no	0.32	-0.14	0.25	-0.02	-0.27
Does sitting help your pain — yes	-1.12	-0.07	-0.14	1.17	-0.18
Does sitting help your pain — no	0.20	0.02	0.04	-0.63	0.05
Does walking help your pain — yes	1.00	-0.31	0.37	-2.04	-0.48
Does walking help your pain — no	-0.36	0.08	-0.12	0.23	0.10
Does lying on face help your pain — yes	0.52	-0.51	1.20	-0.46	-0.54
Does lying on face help your pain — no	-0.09	0.07	-0.36	0.06	0.07
Does sitting make your pain worse — yes	0.22	0.00	0.24	-1.30	0.15
Does sitting make your pain worse — no	-0.25	0.00	-0.30	0.62	-0.16
Does walking make your pain worse — yes	-1.66	-0.12	0.51	0.96	0.04
Does walking make your pain worse — no	0.48	0.06	-0.43	-1.22	-0.03
Does bending make your pain worse — yes	-0.10	0.29	-0.08	-0.35	-0.13
Does bending make your pain worse — no	0.12	-0.40	0.10	0.35	0.16
Does coughing make your pain worse — yes	-0.43	-0.04	0.95	-0.67	0.17
Does coughing make your pain worse — no	0.07	0.01	-0.32	0.10	-0.03
Is your walking distance less than 100 yards — yes	-1.63	-0.69	0.15	1.59	0.25

Table 12.3 Cont

Question	Type				
	1	2	3	4	5
Is your walking distance less than 100 yards — no	0.16	0.11	-0.03	-0.59	-0.05
If walking forces you to stop do you have to sit down — yes	0.00	-0.92	0.46	2.28	-0.13
If walking forces you to stop do you have to sit down — no	0.13	0.08	-0.06	-0.60	0.01
When walking and the pain gets worse is it worse in back — yes	0.04	0.33	-0.90	-0.26	0.15
When walking and the pain gets worse is it worse in back — no	-0.15	-1.54	1.33	0.69	-0.63
When walking and the pain gets worse is it worse in calves — yes	0.00	-0.68	1.22	-0.04	0.08
When walking and the pain gets worse is it worse in calves — no	0.45	0.31	-2.17	0.02	-0.04
When walking do you get numbness or weakness in your legs — yes	-1.59	-0.16	0.63	0.95	0.01
When walking do you get numbness or weakness in your legs — no	0.32	0.06	-0.36	-0.63	0.00
Present pain worse at night — yes	-0.71	-0.12	0.51	-0.78	0.71
Present pain worse at night — no	0.12	0.03	-0.15	0.12	-0.20
Pain about the same throughout the day — yes	-0.50	0.10	0.07	0.43	-0.07
Pain about the same throughout the day — no	0.31	-0.08	-0.06	-0.49	0.05
When your pain first started did you feel a click — yes	-0.02	0.22	-0.52	-0.51	0.11
When your pain first started did you feel a click — no	-0.03	-0.03	0.29	0.24	-0.24
When the pain first started did sitting make it less — yes	-0.24	-0.19	-1.38	1.01	-0.07
When the pain first started did sitting make it less — no	0.05	0.04	0.16	-0.37	0.02
When the pain first started did walking make it less — yes	1.19	-0.44	-0.22	-1.47	-0.38
When the pain first started did walking make it less — no	-0.22	0.06	0.03	0.11	0.04
When the pain first started did sitting make it worse — yes	0.23	-0.16	0.33	-1.11	0.27
When the pain first started did sitting make it worse — no	-0.26	0.15	-0.44	0.57	-0.32
When the pain first started was it worse at night — yes	-0.15	0.18	-0.59	-1.83	0.56
When the pain first started was it worse at night — no	0.03	-0.04	0.09	0.17	-0.14
If your pain has changed since onset is it a different sort — yes	-0.05	-0.37	1.00	-0.28	0.06
If your pain has changed since onset is it a different sort — no	0.02	0.15	-0.92	0.10	-0.03
If your pain has spread since onset has it spread to calves — yes	-1.12	-0.48	1.16	0.45	-0.10
If your pain has spread since onset has it spread to calves — no	0.35	0.23	-1.97	-0.31	0.05
Work started of your first pain — yes	-0.04	0.15	0.67	-0.53	-0.32
Work started of your first pain — no	0.01	-0.06	-0.43	0.16	0.11

Table 12.4 Ranked weights of evidence for facet syndrome (Type 1). Positive values indicate evidence supporting the diagnosis, negative values indicate evidence against the diagnosis

Question	Weight
When the pain first started did walking make it less — yes	1.19
Does walking help your pain — yes	1.00
Is the reason for you coming here leg pain — no	0.55
Does lying on face help your pain — yes	0.52
Does walking make your pain worse — no	0.48
When walking and the pain gets worse is it worse in calves — no	0.45
Is your present pain worst in your legs or feet — yes	0.41
If your pain has spread since onset has it spread to calves — no	0.35
Is your pain intermittent — no	0.32
When walking do you get numbness or weakness in your legs — no	0.32
Pain about the same throughout the day — no	0.31
When the pain first started did sitting make it worse — yes	0.23
Does sitting make your pain worse — yes	0.22
Does sitting help your pain — no	0.20
Is your walking distance less than 100 yards — no	0.16
If walking forces you to stop do you have to sit down — no	0.13
Does bending make your pain worse — no	0.12
Present pain worse at night — no	0.12
Is the reason for you coming here arm or hand pain — no	0.10
Does coughing make your pain worse — no	0.07
When the pain first started did sitting make it less — no	0.05
Is the reason for you coming here back pain — yes	0.04
When walking and the pain gets worse is it worse in back — yes	0.04
When the pain first started was it worse at night — no	0.03
If your pain has changed since onset is it a different sort — no	0.02
Work started of your first pain — no	0.01
Is the reason for you coming here back pain — no	0.00
If walking forces you to stop do you have to sit down — yes	0.00
If your present pain the same severity in your legs and back — no	0.00
When walking and the pain gets worse is it worse in calves — yes	0.00
When your pain first started did you feel a click — yes	−0.02
When the pain first started did you feel a click — no	−0.03
Work started of your first pain — yes	−0.04
If your pain has changed since onset is it a different sort — yes	−0.05
Does lying on face help your pain — no	−0.09
Does bending make your pain worse — yes	−0.10
When walking and the pain gets worse is it worse in back — no	0.15
When the pain first started was it worse at night — yes	−0.15
Is your present pain worst in your back — yes	−0.20
When the pain first started did walking make it less — no	−0.22
When the pain first started did sitting make it less — yes	−0.24
Does sitting make your pain worse — no	−0.25
When the pain first started did sitting make it worse — no	−0.26
Does walking help your pain — no	−0.36
Does coughing make your pain worse — yes	−0.43

Table 12.4   Cont.

Question	Weight
Pain about the same throughout the day — yes	−0.50
Present pain worse at night — yes	−0.71
Is the reason for you coming here leg pain — yes	−1.00
Is your pain continuous — yes	−1.01
Is the reason for you coming here arm or hand pain — yes	−1.03
Does sitting help your pain — yes	−1.12
If your pain has spread since onset has it spread to calves — yes	−1.12
When walking do you get numbness or weakness in your legs — yes	−1.59
Is your walking distance less than 100 yards — yes	−1.63
Does walking make your pain worse — yes	−1.66

Table 12.5   Ranked weights of evidence for discogenic syndrome (Type 2). Positive values indicate evidence supporting the diagnosis, negative values indicate evidence against the diagnosis

Question	Weight
Is your present pain worst in your back — yes	0.66
When walking and the pain gets worse is it worse in back — yes	0.33
When walking and the pain gets worse is it worse in calves — no	0.31
Is your pain continuous — yes	0.29
Does bending make your pain worse — yes	0.29
If your pain has spread since onset has it spread to calves — no	0.23
When your pain first started did you feel a click — yes	0.22
Is the reason for you coming here leg pain — no	0.21
When the pain first started was it worse at night — yes	0.18
When the pain first started did sitting make it worse — no	0.15
If your pain has changed since onset is it a different sort — no	0.15
Work stated of your first pain — yes	0.15
If your walking distance less than 100 yards — no	0.11
Is your present pain the same severity in your legs and back — no	0.10
Pain about the same throughout the day — yes	0.10
Does walking help your pain — no	0.08
If walking forces you to stop do you have to sit down — no	0.08
Does lying on face help your pain — no	0.07
When walking do you get numbness or weakness in your legs — no	0.06
Is the reason for you coming here arm or hand pain — no	0.06
Does walking make your pain worse — no	0.06
When the pain first started did walking make it less — no	0.06
Is the reason for you coming here back pain — yes	0.04
When the pain first started did sitting make it less — no	0.04
Present pain worse at night — no	0.03
Does sitting help your pain — no	0.02
Does coughing make your pain worse — no	0.01
Does sitting make your pain worse — yes	0.00
Does sitting make your pain worse — no	0.00

Table 12.5   Cont.

Question	Weight
When the pain first started did you feel a click — no	−0.03
Does coughing make your pain worse — yes	−0.04
When the pain first started was it worse at night — no	−0.04
Work started of your first pain — no	−0.06
Does sitting help your pain — yes	−0.07
Pain about the same throughout the day — no	−0.08
Does walking make your pain worse — yes	−0.12
Present pain worse at night — yes	−0.12
Is your pain intermittent — no	−0.14
When walking do you get numbness or weakness in your legs — yes	−0.16
When the pain first started did sitting make it worse — yes	−0.16
When the pain first started did sitting make it less — yes	−0.19
Is the reason for you coming here leg pain — yes	−0.25
Does walking help your pain — yes	−0.31
If your pain has changed since onset is it a different sort — yes	−0.37
Does bending make your pain worse — no	−0.40
When the pain first started did walking make it less — yes	−0.44
Is the reason for you coming here arm or hand pain — yes	−0.48
If your pain has spread since onset has it spread to calves — yes	−0.48
Does lying on face help your pain — yes	−0.51
When walking and the pain gets worse is it worse in calves — yes	−0.68
Is your walking distance less than 100 yards — yes	−0.69
If walking forces you to stop do you have to sit down — yes	−0.92
Is your present pain worst in your legs or feet — yes	−1.03
When walking and the pain gets worse is it worse in back — no	−1.54
Is the reason for you coming here back pain — no	−1.86

Table 12.6   Ranked weights of evidence for discogenic and root compression syndrome (Type 3). Positive values indicate evidence supporting the diagnosis, negative values indicate evidence against the diagnosis

Question	Weight
Is the reason for you coming here back pain — no	2.18
When walking and the pain gets worse is it worse in back — no	1.33
When walking and the pain gets worse is it worse in calves — yes	1.22
Does lying on face help your pain — yes	1.20
If your pain has spread since onset has it spread to calves — yes	1.16
Is your present pain worst in your legs or feet — yes	1.10
If your pain has changed since onset is it a different sort — yes	1.00
Does coughing make your pain worse — yes	0.95
Is the reason for you coming here leg pain — yes	0.67
Work started of your first pain — yes	0.67
When walking do you get numbness or weakness in your legs — yes	0.63
Does walking make your pain worse — yes	0.51
Present pain worse at night — yes	0.51

Table 12.6   Cont

Question	Weight
If walking forces you to stop do you have to sit down — yes	0.46
Does walking help your pain — yes	0.37
When the pain first started did sitting make it worse — yes	0.33
When the pain first started did you feel a click — no	0.29
Is your pain intermittent — no	0.25
Does sitting make your pain worse — yes	0.24
When the pain first started did sitting make it less — no	0.16
Is your walking distance less than 100 yards — yes	0.15
Does bending make your pain worse — no	0.10
Is the reason for you coming here arm or hand pain — no	0.09
When the pain first started was it worse at night — no	0.09
Pain about the same throughout the day — yes	0.07
Does sitting help your pain — no	0.04
When the pain first started did walking make it less — no	0.03
Is your present pain the same severity in your legs and back — no	0.00
Is your walking distance less than 100 yards — no	−0.03
If walking forces you to stop do you have to sit down — no	−0.06
Pain about the same throughout the day — no	−0.06
Does bending make your pain worse — yes	−0.08
Does walking help your pain — no	−0.12
Does sitting help your pain — yes	−0.14
Present pain worse at night — no	−0.15
Is the reason for you coming here back pain — yes	−0.19
When the pain first started did walking make it less — yes	−0.22
Does sitting make your pain worse — no	−0.30
Does coughing make your pain worse — no	−0.32
When walking do you get numbness or weakness in your legs — no	−0.36
Does lying on face help your pain — no	−0.36
Does walking make your pain worse — no	−0.43
Work started of your first pain — no	−0.43
When the pain first started did sitting make it worse — no	−0.44
When your pain first started did you feel a click — yes	−0.52
When the pain first started was it worse at night — yes	−0.59
Is your pain continuous — yes	−0.85
When walking and the pain gets worse is it worse in back — yes	−0.90
If your pain has changed since onset is it a different sort — no	−0.92
Is the reason for you coming here arm or hand pain — yes	−0.97
Is the reason for you coming here leg pain — no	−1.37
When the pain first started did sitting make it less — yes	−1.38
If your pain has spread since onset has it spread to calves — no	−1.97
Is your present pain worst in your back — yes	−2.04
When walking and the pain gets worse is it worse in calves — no	−2.17

Table 12.7 Ranked weights of evidence for neurogenic claudication syndrome (Type 4). Positive values indicate evidence supporting the diagnosis, negative values indicate evidence against the diagnosis

Question	Weight
If walking forces you to stop do you have to sit down — yes	2.28
Is your walking distance less than 100 yards — yes	1.59
Is the reason for you coming here back pain — no	1.21
Does sitting help your pain — yes	1.17
When the pain first started did sitting make it less — yes	1.01
Does walking make your pain worse — yes	0.96
When walking do you get numbness or weakness in your legs — yes	0.95
When walking and the pain gets worse is it worse in back — no	0.69
Does sitting make your pain worse — no	0.62
Is your present pain the same severity in your legs and back — no	0.58
When the pain first started did sitting make it worse — no	0.57
Is the reason for you coming here leg pain — yes	0.53
Is the reason for you coming here arm or hand pain — yes	0.45
If your pain has spread since onset has it spread to calves — yes	0.45
Pain about the same throughout the day — yes	0.43
Does bending make your pain worse — no	0.35
Is your present pain worst in your legs or feet — yes	0.34
When the pain first started did you feel a click — no	0.24
Does walking help your pain — no	0.23
When the pain first started was it worse at night — no	0.17
Work started of your first pain — no	0.16
Present pain worse at night — no	0.12
When the pain first started did walking make it less — no	0.11
Does coughing make your pain worse — no	0.10
If your pain has changed since onset is it a different sort — no	0.10
Does lying on face help your pain — no	0.06
Is your pain continuous — yes	0.05
When walking and the pain gets worse is it worse in calves — no	0.02
Is your pain intermittent — no	−0.02
When walking and the pain gets worse is it worse in calves — yes	−0.04
Is the reason for you coming here back pain — yes	−0.07
Is the reason for you coming here arm or hand pain — no	−0.07
When walking and the pain gets worse is it worse in back — yes	−0.26
If your pain has changed since onset is it a different sort — yes	−0.28
If your pain has spread since onset has it spread to calves — no	−0.31
Does bending make your pain worse — yes	−0.35
When the pain first started did sitting make it less — no	−0.37
Does lying on face help your pain — yes	−0.46
Pain about the same throughout the day — no	−0.49
When your pain first started did you feel a click — yes	−0.51
Is your present pain worst in your back — yes	−0.52
Work started to your first pain — yes	−0.53
Is your walking distance less than 100 yards — no	−0.59
If walking forces you to stop do you have to sit down — no	−0.60
When walking do you get numbness or weakness in your legs — no	−0.63

Table 12.7   Cont

Question	Weight
Does sitting help your pain — no	−0.63
Does coughing make your pain worse — yes	−0.67
Is the reason for you coming here leg pain — no	−0.76
Present pain worse at night — yes	−0.78
When the pain first started did sitting make it worse — yes	−1.11
Does walking make your pain worse — no	−1.22
Does sitting make your pain worse — yes	−1.30
When the pain first started did walking make it less — yes	−1.47
When the pain first started was it worse at night — yes	−1.83
Does walking help your pain — yes	−2.04

Table 12.8   Ranked weights of evidence for unclassifiable syndrome (Type 5). Positive values indicate evidence supporting the diagnosis, negative values indicate evidence against the diagnosis

Question	Weight
Is the reason for you coming here arm or hand pain — yes	1.07
Present pain worse at night — yes	0.71
When the pain first started was it worse at night — yes	0.56
Is your pain continuous — yes	0.46
Is your present pain the same severity in your legs and back — no	0.39
Is the reason for you coming here leg pain — yes	0.31
When the pain first started did sitting make it worse — yes	0.27
Is your walking distance less than 100 yards — yes	0.25
Does coughing make your pain worse — yes	0.17
Does bending make your pain worse — no	0.16
Does sitting make your pain worse — yes	0.15
When walking and the pain gets worse is it worse in back — yes	0.15
When your pain first started did you feel a click — yes	0.11
Work started of your first pain — no	0.11
Does walking help your pain — no	0.10
When walking and the pain gets worse is it worse in calves — yes	0.08
Does lying on face help your pain — no	0.07
If your pain has changed since onset is it a different sort — yes	0.06
Does sitting help your pain — no	0.05
Pain about the same throughout the day — no	0.05
If your pain has spread since onset has it spread to calves — no	0.05
Is your present pain worst in your back — yes	0.04
Does walking make your pain worse — yes	0.04
When the pain first started did walking make it less — no	0.04
Is the reason for you coming here back pain — no	0.02
When the pain first started did sitting make it less — no	0.02
When walking do you get numbness or weakness in your legs — yes	0.01
If walking forces you to stop do you have to sit down — no	0.01

Table 12.8   Cont

Question	Weight
Is the reason for you coming here back pain — yes	0.00
When walking do you get numbness or weakness in your legs — no	0.00
Does walking make your pain worse — no	−0.03
Does coughing make your pain worse — no	−0.03
If your pain has changed since onset is it a different sort — no	−0.03
When walking and the pain gets worse is it worse in calves — no	−0.04
Is your walking distance less than 100 yards — no	−0.05
Pain about the same throughout the day — yes	−0.07
When the pain first started did sitting make it less — yes	−0.07
If your pain has spread since onset has it spread to calves — yes	−0.10
Does bending make your pain worse — yes	−0.13
If walking forces you to stop do you have to sit down — yes	−0.13
When the pain first started was it worse at night — no	−0.14
Does sitting make your pain worse — no	−0.16
Does sitting help your pain — yes	−0.18
Is the reason for you coming here arm or hand pain — no	−0.20
Present pain worse at night — no	−0.20
When the pain first started did you feel a click — no	−0.24
Is your pain intermittent — no	−0.27
Is your present pain worst in your legs or feet — yes	−0.31
When the pain first started did sitting make it worse — no	−0.32
Work started of your first pain — yes	−0.32
Is the reason for you coming here leg pain — no	−0.33
When the pain first started did walking make it less — yes	−0.38
Does walking help your pain — yes	−0.48
Does lying on face help your pain — yes	−0.54
When walking and the pain gets worse is it worse in back — no	−0.63

classification performed here used more than the clinical data obtained at the computer interview. Information from physical examination, investigative procedures, and response to treatment was used. We have defined the features of a history that a surgeon used to classify a group of patients into syndromes that were felt to reflect pathology. This is a task that most clinicians find difficult.

This technique provides a powerful method of defining the contents of a clinical syndrome as it is understood by an individual clinician. It is clear that there is considerable difficulty in communicating the contents of one clinician's perceptions of a clinical syndrome to another. Different users of this computer interview system can use the database to define these differences more clearly to one another, assuming that all the patient populations respond to the computer interview system in a similar manner. We promote this technique as one which will help to overcome these difficulties. The data derived from this technique could be used to develop

Table 12.9 Simple weights of evidence for five group classification of back pain ordered by range. The highest range indicates the most discriminating question

Question	Types					Range
	1	2	3	4	5	
Is the reason for you coming here back pain — no	0.00	−1.86	2.18	1.21	0.02	4.04
Is your walking distance less than 100 yards — yes	−1.63	−0.69	0.15	1.59	0.25	3.22
If walking forces you to stop do you have to sit down — yes	0.00	−0.92	0.46	2.28	−0.13	3.2
Does walking help your pain — yes	1.00	−0.31	0.37	−2.04	−0.48	3.04
When walking and the pain gets worse is it worse in back — no	−0.15	−1.54	1.33	0.69	−0.63	2.87
Is your present pain worst in your back — yes	−0.20	0.66	−2.04	−0.52	0.04	2.7
When the pain first started did walking make it less — yes	1.19	−0.44	−0.22	−1.47	−0.38	2.66
When walking and the pain gets worse is it worse in calves — no	0.45	0.31	−2.17	0.02	−0.04	2.62
Does walking make your pain worse — yes	−1.66	−0.12	0.51	0.96	0.04	2.62
When walking do you get numbness or weakness in your legs — yes	−1.59	−0.16	0.63	0.95	0.01	2.54
When the pain first started was it worse at night — yes	−0.15	0.18	−0.59	−1.83	0.56	2.39
When the pain first started did sitting make it less — yes	−0.24	−0.19	−1.38	1.01	−0.07	2.39
If your pain has spread since onset has it spread to calves — no	0.35	0.23	−1.97	−0.31	0.05	2.32
Does sitting help your pain — yes	−1.12	−0.07	−0.14	1.17	−0.18	2.29
If your pain has spread since onset has it spread to calves — yes	−1.12	−0.48	1.16	0.45	−0.10	2.28
Is your present pain worst in your legs or feet — yes	0.41	−1.03	1.10	0.34	−0.31	2.13
Is the reason for you coming here arm or hand pain — yes	−1.03	−0.48	−0.97	0.45	1.07	2.1
Is the reason for you coming here leg pain — no	0.55	0.21	−1.37	−0.76	−0.33	1.92
When walking and the pain gets worse is it worse in calves — yes	0.00	−0.68	1.22	−0.04	0.08	1.9
Does lying on face help your pain — yes	0.52	−0.51	1.20	−0.46	−0.54	1.74
Does walking make your pain worse — no	0.48	0.06	−0.43	−1.22	−0.03	1.7
Is the reason for you coming here leg pain — yes	−1.00	−0.25	0.67	0.53	0.31	1.67
Does coughing make your pain worse — yes	−0.43	−0.04	0.95	−0.67	0.17	1.62
Does sitting make your pain worse — yes	0.22	0.00	0.24	−1.30	0.15	1.54
Present pain worse at night — yes	−0.71	−0.12	0.51	−0.78	0.71	1.49
Is your pain continuous — yes	−1.01	0.29	−0.85	0.05	0.46	1.47
When the pain first started did sitting make it worse — yes	0.23	−0.16	0.33	−1.11	0.27	1.44

Question						
If your pain has changed since onset is it a different sort — yes	-0.05	-0.37	1.00	-0.28	0.06	1.37
When walking and the pain gets worse is it worse in back — yes	0.04	0.33	-0.90	-0.26	0.15	1.23
Work started of your first pain — yes	-0.04	0.15	0.67	-0.53	-0.32	1.2
If your pain has changed since onset is it a different sort — no	0.02	0.15	-0.92	0.10	-0.03	1.07
When the pain first started did sitting make it worse — no	-0.26	0.15	-0.44	0.57	-0.32	1.01
When walking do you get numbness or weakness in your legs — no	0.32	0.06	-0.36	-0.63	0.00	0.95
Pain about the same throughout the day — yes	-0.50	0.10	0.07	0.43	-0.07	0.93
Does sitting make your pain worse — no	-0.25	0.00	-0.30	0.62	-0.16	0.92
Does sitting help your pain — no	0.20	0.02	0.04	-0.63	0.05	0.83
Pain about the same throughout the day — no	0.31	-0.08	-0.06	-0.49	0.05	0.8
Is your walking distance less than 100 yards — no	0.16	0.11	-0.03	-0.59	-0.05	0.75
Does bending make your pain worse — no	0.12	-0.40	0.10	0.35	0.16	0.75
When your pain first started did you feel a click — yes	-0.02	0.22	-0.52	-0.51	0.11	0.74
If walking forces you to stop do you have to sit down — no	0.13	0.08	-0.06	-0.60	0.01	0.73
Does bending make your pain worse — yes	-0.10	0.29	-0.08	-0.35	-0.13	0.64
Work started of your first pain — no	0.01	-0.06	-0.43	0.16	0.11	0.59
Is your pain intermittent — no	0.32	-0.14	0.25	-0.02	-0.27	0.59
Does walking help your pain — no	-0.36	0.08	-0.12	0.23	0.10	0.59
Is your present pair the same severity in your legs and back — no	0.00	0.10	0.00	0.58	0.39	0.58
When the pain first started did you feel a click — no	-0.03	-0.03	0.29	0.24	-0.24	0.53
When the pain first started did sitting make it less — no	0.05	0.04	0.16	-0.37	0.02	0.53
Does lying on face help your pain — no	-0.09	0.07	-0.36	0.06	0.07	0.43
Does coughing make your pain worse — no	0.07	0.01	-0.32	0.10	-0.03	0.42
When the pain first started did walking make it less — no	-0.22	0.06	0.03	0.11	0.04	0.33
Present pain worse at night — no	0.12	0.03	-0.15	0.12	-0.20	0.32
When the pain first started was it worse at night — no	0.03	-0.04	0.09	0.17	-0.14	0.31
Is the reason for you coming here arm or hand pain — no	0.10	0.06	0.09	-0.07	-0.20	0.3
Is the reason for you coming here back pain — yes	0.04	0.04	-0.19	-0.07	0.00	0.23

a computer-based expert system to distribute patients into diagnostic groups.

We are pleased to provide the software of our interview system to other interested users in return for data defining the diagnostic categories into which the user feels his or her patients fall. It is then relatively straightforward to analyse their classification in a similar manner. In the absence of specific diagnostic tests for specific syndromes, this is one method by which the classification of this obscure symptom may be clarified.

A summary of the important features of the syndromes recognised by JCTF is as follows:

- *Type 1*: A young patient with occasional leg pain (but not below the knees) eased by walking and lying on the face and sometimes aggravated by sitting. The pain is unlikely to be continuous and there is rarely leg numbness or walking symptoms.

- *Type 2*: A patient with continuous back pain. If leg pain is present it is not as severe as the back pain. If the pain is aggravated by walking it is the back pain that gets worse. Walking distance is however rarely less than 100 yards. Bending tends to make the pain worse and there is occasionally a 'click' with onset.

- *Type 3*: A patient with a predominant complaint of leg pain that may be aggravated by walking. The pain has often spread into the calves since the onset of symptoms. The pain may be eased by lying on the face and aggravated by coughing. The pain is rarely eased by sitting and unlikely to be continuous.

- *Type 4*: An older patient with a predominance of leg symptoms (pain, sensory and motor changes) related to walking and eased by sitting. There may be some back pain and the pain has often spread to the calves since onset. The pain is unlikely to be worse at night. There is a likely to be associated arm and hand pain.

- *Type 5*: A patient with continuous pain often in the back and legs in equal severity. They are very likely to complain of arm and neck pain. The pain is often worse at night and may be aggravated by walking but there is unlikely to be any associated numbness or weakness.

References

Fairbank, J. C. T. and Hall, H. (1990). History taking and physical examination, identification of syndromes of back pain. In: *The Lumbar Spine* eds. J. Weinstein & S. Weisel. WB Sauaders & Co., Philadelphia.

Knill-Jones, R. P. (1987). Logic in medicine, *British Medical Journal*, 295, 1392–6.
Macartney, F.J. (1987). Diagnostic logic, *British Medical Journal*, **295**, 1325–31.
Pynsent, P. B. & Fairbank, J. C. T. (1989). Computer interview system for patients with back pain, *Journal of Biomedical Engineering*, **11**, 25–9.
Thomas, A. M. C., Fairbank, J. C. T., Pynsent, P. B. & Baker, D. J. (1989). A computer-based interview system for patients with back pain: A validation study, *Spine*, **14**, 844–6.

Discussion

Burton: Can you tell us anything at all about the cause of symptoms? You have defined some groups for us, but what can we expect from these groups?

Fairbank (in reply): We still do not know that. That would be another study. We have been looking at the time scale of disability in these patients. The real reason for presenting this is to show to those people using our interview system that this is a way of using our database for analysing the way that they divide up their patients. It gives us some idea of what each one of the doctors are talking about. If, say, in Nottingham, Bob Mulholland is looking at patients, and he uses ten different types, or maybe five types, but they are slightly different from mine, we can actually get an idea whether we are talking about the same groups or not.

I am not saying that this is the way to classify back pain, but it happens to be a convenient clinical system which I use. We have all got systems as we have heard this morning. What it does is pull out the features of real live patients.

Macdonald: When you did your original study, you differentiated patients into 'responders' and 'non-responders'; your non-responders, if I remember correctly, included people who went on to show that they had disc-produced sciatica? So the responders and non-responders differentiation you used was not just within, shall we say, a diagnosis of non-specific back pain, but it included a whole range of patients.

Fairbank: That particular study was carried out on people with their first attack of back pain, and these patients were a cross section of patients referred to me by GPs. What I am saying is that this study influenced my thinking, although there were only a small number of patients. When we looked at the 'responders' and 'non-responders' to the intra-facet injections, there were a few clear-cut clinical features which distinguished the two groups. Walking, for instance, was an important exacerbating or relieving factor.

Fairbank, J. C. T., Park, W. M., McCall, I. M. & O'Brien, J. P. (1981). Apophyseal injections of local anaesthetic as a diagnostic aid in low back syndromes, *Spine*, **6**, 598–601.

Macdonald: What did you think of the recent paper in *Spine* (Murtagh, 1988), showing that you are very likely to find, with an intra-facet local anaesthetic injection of more than 2 ml, that it very quickly ruptures and the agent actually spreads quite widely?

Murtagh F. R. (1988). Computed tomography and fluoroscopy guided anaesthesia and steroid injection in facet syndrome, *Spine*, **13**, 686–9.

Fairbank: I am sure the local anaesthetic diffuses rapidly. This is why I did not like calling patients who responded to the injection sufferers of a facet syndrome but prefered to call them 'responders'. We did discuss it in the original publication. The response may be due to local anaesthetic diffusion, or it may be an 'acupuncture' effect, it may be all sorts of things that one is actually doing to the patient at the time. What it did was to distinguish two clinical groups and I am saying that this study now influences my thinking a bit. I hardly ever use facet-joint injections as a diagnostic technique now.

Unidentified questioner: Have you seen a relation in your rules with X-rays?

Fairbank: We are looking at this at present. I cannot answer this question yet. Experience and previous studies would suggest that their contribution is limited.

13 *D. W. L. Hukins*

Clinical signs and dynamics of segmental instability

13.1 Introduction

The aim of this chapter is to investigate the biomechanical reasons for the clinical signs associated with segmental instability of the spine. Segmental instability has been described in many different ways but few attempts have been made at a precise definition (Nachemson, 1985). Porter (1986) has summarised its signs as 'excessive, unnatural movement'. The manifestation of this unnatural movement when rising from a stooped position could be taken as a clinical definition of instability; it involves jerky movement ('extension catch') and, sometimes, the use of the arms to provide additional support (Porter, 1986). It seems more sensible to define instability in terms of the clinical signs which are observed, rather than by some presumed mechanism, which may or may not be the cause of these symptoms in a particular individual.

Previously the analogy of stable, neutral and unstable equilibrium of a static system has been used to rationalise the mechanics of instability (Pope and Panjabi, 1985). The idea is that, because the normal restraints are lacking, the unstable spine can move inappropriately. However, the signs of instability are associated with movement and are not simply a general laxity of the spine. As we do not move through a series of equilibrium positions, a static model, based on the assumption that at any instant we must adopt a posture which is in equilibrium, cannot be used to analyse movement. Statics is the mechanics of systems at rest; the mechanics of moving systems is called dynamics. In this chapter some simple concepts of dynamics are used to illustrate how jerky movements might occur.

13.2 Dynamics of the spine

Movement occurs as a result of muscular contraction. Contraction of a muscle, or system of muscles, generates a resultant force, F, which leads to a time-dependant change in the position, x, of the body. The relationship between F and x may be represented by:

$$F = a_0 x + a_1 \dot{x} + a_2 \ddot{x} \qquad (1)$$

where $\dot{x}$ is the rate of change of x (velocity), and $\ddot{x}$ is the rate of change of $\dot{x}$ (acceleration). Here a_0 represents the stiffness of the system, a_1 provides a measure of energy dissipation, and a_2 is the inertia. For the present, we may consider that the stiffness arises from the need to stretch joint tissues. The mechanism for energy dissipation is usually considered to be fluid flow in or out of tissues but intrinsic viscoelasticity of tissues could also lead to dissipation of energy. The greater the value of a_1, the greater the energy dissipation by the system. For simple translational motion the inertia is simply the mass of the body. However, a_2 has a more complicated meaning (involving 'moment of inertia') when applied to bending; nevertheless, a_2 is expected to depend on the mass and dimensions of the body. Thus the 'second order' form of equation (1) is the simplest which provides a physically reasonable model for movement of the spine. If a_0, a_1 and a_2 are constant, equation 1 can be solved to show how position, x, depends on time, t (see, for example, Healey, 1975). There are several reasons why a_0 and a_1 are not constant throughout the whole range of movement. Since spinal ligaments do not have a constant stiffness and because different ligaments tend to be stretched at different stages of movement, a_0 and a_1 depend on x. The system is then said to be 'non-linear'. There are insufficient experimental data to begin to analyse the spine as a non-linear system. Even if it were possible, such an analysis would probably disguise many simple ideas by its complexity. Fortunately, a non-linear system can be considered to be linear for sufficiently small displacements although, in the case of the spine, we do not know how small they would have to be.

I have, therefore, used equation (1), with constant values of a_0, a_1 and a_2, to provide a simple model system which illustrates the principles involved in the control of movement. For the purpose of illustration, consider the position of the body at time $t = 0$ to have a postion which is arbitrarily assigned to have $x = 0$. This original posture is changed by the sudden application of a force which moves the body and continues to be applied so as to maintain it in a new posture, arbitrarily assigned a value of $x = 1$. The positions adopted by the body, while it is moving, depend on the value of a damping factor defined by:

$$d = (a_1^2 / 4a_2 a_0)^{\frac{1}{2}} \qquad (2)$$

Figure 13.1 shows how the position, x, depends on time for different values of d. Instead of plotting x against t, this figure shows x plotted against T which is defined by

$$T = 2\pi f_0 \, t \qquad (3)$$

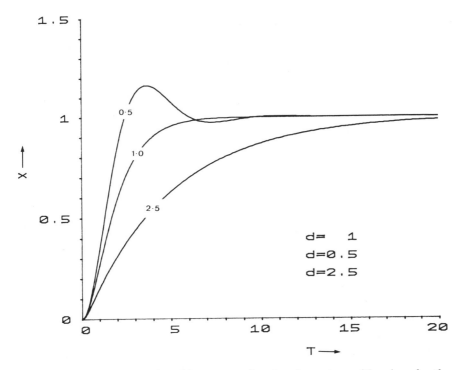

Fig. 13.1 Dependence of position, x, on time for the system with values for the damping factor, d, of 0.5, 1.0 and 2.5. T is related to time, t, by equation (3). The curve with $d = 0.5$ shows the jerky behaviour characteristic of segmental instability

where f_0 is the natural frequency of the system defined by

$$f_0 = (1/2\pi)(a_0/a_2)^{\frac{1}{2}} \tag{4}$$

There is a simple physical interpretation of f_0. In the absence of damping, application of the force would lead the system to oscillate indefinitely; f_0 is then simply the oscillation frequency.

Ideally our model system should be 'critically damped'. A critically damped system has $d = 1$ and moves to the desired position without over-shooting, as shown in Figure 13.1. An 'overdamped' system has a value for $d > 1$ and the desired position may never be attained in the required time scale. This behaviour is illustrated in the figure for a system with $d = 2.5$. However, when $d < 1$ the system does not move smoothly but exhibits the jerky movement associated with segmental instability of the spine. It is then said to be 'underdamped'. In Figure 13.1 this is illustrated by the system having a value of $d = 0.5$. As a result it overshoots in a way associated with extension catch. Lower d values can lead to more extreme jerky behaviour. In segmental instability this behaviour could arise from a low value of a_1, i.e. impairment of energy dissipation mechanisms. The reason is that a_2 depends largely on stature and a_0 is likely to be similar to that for the normal population, since patients demonstrating segmental instability tend to exhibit the normal range of flexion (Porter, 1986). In the terms of dynamics, this jerky system is not 'unstable' because it eventually settles to the same position as the critically damped system. However, the signs of segmental 'instability' are those which are associated with an underdamped system.

13.3 **Implications**

There are several ways in which the energy dissipation mechanisms of the intervertebral joint could be impaired – leading to the signs of segmental instability. Mechanical derangement of the joint, as in spondylolisthesis, may mean that it can be moved without its tissues being strained as normal. Energy dissipation mechanisms associated with tissue strain (e.g. fluid flow; Maroudas, 1980) will then be reduced. Disc degeneration is associated with a reduction in its fluid content (Lyons *et al.*, 1981; Stevens *et al.*, 1982). Degenerate discs may then be inadequately hydrated for fluid to be expressed. Both spondylolisthesis and disc degeneration have been listed as being associated with instability (Nelson, 1987).

However, the healthy body can damp its movements actively, by contraction of opposing muscles, as well as passively, by the response of its connective tissues. Muscles may then be used to compensate for an inadequate passive response in the connective tissues. The muscular hypertrophy and fatigue when standing, which may be associated with instability (Porter, 1986), suggest that at least some of these patients place more than usual reliance on their muscles to maintain posture. Conversely, neurological problems which lead to impairment of muscular coordination might give rise to the signs of instability because poor coordination would lead to perturbed active damping. In either case, holding the legs when rising from a stooped position provides an additional control mechanism.

Acknowledgements

I thank Drs R. M. Aspden and S. Lees for discussion.

References

Healey, M. (1975). *Principles of Automatic Control*. Hodder and Stoughton, London.
Lyons, G., Eisenstein, S. M. and Sweet, M. B. E. (1981). Biochemical changes in intervertebral disc degeneration, *Biochimica et Biophysica Acta*, **673**, 443–53.

Maroudas, A. (1980). Physical chemistry of articular cartilage and intervertebral disc. In: *The Joints and Synovial Fluid*, vol. 2, ed. L. Sokoloff, pp. 240–93. Academic Press, New York.

Nachemson, A. (1985). Lumbar spine instability, *Spine*, **10**, 290–1.

Nelson, M. A. (1987). Indications for spinal surgery in low back pain. In: *The Lumbar Spine and Back Pain*, 3rd Edn., ed. M. I. V. Jayson, pp. 321–52. Churchill Livingstone, London.

Pope, M. H. and Panjabi, M. (1985). Biomechanical definitions of spinal instability, *Spine*, **10**, 255–6.

Porter, R. W. (1986). *Management of Back Pain*, Churchill Livingstone, Edinburgh.

Stevens, R. L., Ryvar, R., Robertson, W. R., O'Brien, J. P. and Beard, H. K. (1982). Biological changes in the annulus fibrosus in patients with low back pain, *Spine*, **7**, 223–33.

Discussion

Fairbank: How are we going to measure this wobbliness? There have been many studies of lumbar spine motion and yet, so far, no one has come up with an ideal system.

Hukins (in reply): In principle, it could be measured by a displacement, velocity or acceleration transducer whose frequency response included the frequencies to be measured. A range of designs for such transducers is available (Cobbold, 1974). It should also be possible to make such measurements from video recordings, for which the standard image acquisition rate is effectively 25 Hz, given that there are simple computer techniques for making dimensional measurements from video recordings (Aspden *et al.*, 1988).

Aspden, R. M., Gleave, B. D. and Hukins, D. W. L. (1988). Dimensional measurements on images from a video camera or cassette recorder using a BBC microcomputer, *Journal of Biomedical Engineering*, **10**, 291–1.

Cobbold R. S. C. (1974). *Transducers for Biomedical Measurements: Principles and Applications*, pp. 114–89, Wiley, London.

Nelson: Are you satisfied that Richard Porter's definition is going to help? Does erratic movement occur in someone who is recovering from an abdominal operation or who has had some sort of illness in which the spine as a structure is stable, but is wobbly because the muscle is controlling it inadequately. I feel that this definition is only part of what I think must be a more detailed description which common instability would encompass. I am worried that you may be following a red herring.

Hukins (in reply): There is no doubt that it is difficult to define 'instability' and that there are many different definitions. Indeed, there seems to be no consensus in the literature as to what the term is intended to include.

Consequently, I have taken one clear definition which is based on observable clinical signs. I have then tried to find how these signs could be accounted for in terms of the biomechanics of the spine.

I agree that the behaviour of the muscles controlling the spine has to be taken into account and have discussed this briefly at the end of my paper. Furthermore, the abdominal muscles and intra-abdominal pressure are expected to have a direct influence on spinal mechanics (Aspden, 1987). When considering motion and, therefore, instability, the spine has to be considered as part of the whole body.

The simple model described at the beginning of my pager is clearly inadequate to deal with all the problems involved. It is intended simply as a way of showing the kind of approach which is needed for a biomechanical analysis of instability as defined in terms of movement.

Aspden, R. M. (1987). Intra-abdominal pressure and its role in spinal mechanics, *Clinical Biomechanics*, **2**, 168–74.

Helliwell: Could you not put your patients on an electro-mechanical shaker and measure the frequency response of the spine?

Hukins (in reply): I would be concerned about shaking patients with back pain. Furthermore, the large amplitude oscilliations which are induced on a shaker would be difficult to analyse in order to learn about the dynamics of the spine. The reason is that the system would be 'non-linear' for the reasons I discussed.

Helliwell: I am working with James Smeathers in Leeds, and we actually had people walking up and down which gave us a much more pure input than shaking people.

Hukins (in reply): I am sure that this is a much more natural way of assessing motion. I do not know whether it could tell us much about instability or the dynamics of the spine.

Hammond: Can you not look at segmental instability using dynamic radiography in flexion, extension and lateral flexion. Quite often a late retrolisthesis or late lateral listhesis is demonstable on an extension or torsion film that does now show on plain films.

Hukins (in reply): Yes, I am sure you could were that the only cause of instability.

Hammond: I am saying I was looking for instances of instability on a routine basis.

Pearcy: Just to comment on that, Ian Stokes in Vermont has used a three-dimensional X-ray system to examine patients with clinically diagnosed 'instability' of the L4/5 level, and has found very little evidence of abnormal motion.

Stokes, I. A. F. & Frymoyer, J. W. (1987). Segmental motion and instability, *Spine*, **12**, 688–91.

Nargolwala: Although one can demonstrate radiologically, or by any other sophisticated methods, the segmental instability (by this I mean abnormal erratic or excessive movement of one vertebra on another), I think all of us have experienced patients where they do not always produce symptoms. On the other hand, even in minor instability can produce a lot of symptoms. I wonder if you have any ideas about a clinical reason why this happens?

Hukins (in reply): I have been concerned with instability defined in terms of clinical signs, rather than some radiological observation which is supposed to be associated with instability. If the patient has no symptoms, it is difficult to understand how the spine could be considered unstable.

Nargolwala: The question was, assuming that you prove that there is erratic motion, would it always produce the symptoms?

Hukins (in reply): There is no necessary reason for associating erratic motion with pain.

Pain-provoking clinical tests as prognostic indicators in low back trouble: a basis for classification?

14.1 Introduction

Low back pain is a symptom which may be caused by a variety of diseases and disorders of the lumbar region, only some of which are presently identifiable; the underlying cause of pain and disability in most instances of low back trouble (LBT) being unknown (Jayson, 1970). The whole spectrum of LBT poses a serious problem of classification (Anderson, 1977), and furthermore different disciplines, for example biomechanics and epidemiology, may well have different needs from a system of classification; it is only through scientific research that useful classification or diagnostic categories of LBT will emerge which can form the basis for a rational choice of treatment (Weber & Burton, 1986).

Although most episodes of LBT seem to resolve within 3 months of onset (Horal, 1969), recurrence is common within a year (Troup *et al.*, 1981). Lankhorst *et al.* (1982) reported symptoms persisting for up to 3 years in spite of therapeutic intervention. There is a clear clinical advantage if a chronic course of symptoms could be predicted at presentation. Patients requiring special care (or further investigation) could be identified early, whilst those likely to have a short symptomatic course could be reassured.

When a specific pathology can be identified objectively (e.g. radiographically), a classification within that pathological disorder is possible. For instance, Wiltse *et al.* (1976) classified spondylolysis and spondylolisthesis into five categories, although it should be remembered that these conditions can also occur in the symptom-free (La Rocca & Macnab, 1969).

In the absence of diagnostic categories with a known pathophysiology it has been suggested that homogenous groups of LBT patients should be determined with respect to the temporal pattern of symptoms (Weber &

Burton, 1986). A clinical application of this approach would be a classification based on the symptomatic state at, say, 3 months and 1 year from presentation. The predictive criteria of such a classification should be based on simple clinical data. Classifications based on symptom patterns and results from clinical investigations have been described by various workers (Nachemson & Anderson, 1982; Barker, 1977; Mathews *et al.*, 1983; Nelson, 1986), but the temporal aspects of symptoms in these groupings was not the major concern. Sophisticated statistical techniques have been employed to search for clusters of clinical and anamnestic data which may define homogenous groups (Kersley *et al.*, 1978; McQuaid-Korenko *et al.*, 1984; Heinrich *et al.*, 1985), with varying degrees of success; again clinical prediction of short- or long-term outcome was not adequately determined. However, Burton & Getty (1989) have shown general associations between clinical examination findings and the subsequent course of symptoms during the year following presentation in patients with low back trouble.

The object of this work was to test the hypothesis that the 1-year course of LBT symptoms (in the absence of a formal diagnosis) can be predicted by a mathematical model based on responses to pain-provoking clinical tests combined with descriptions of the site of pain.

14.2 Methods

The subjects were 109 LBT patients attending an orthopaedic out-patient department ($n = 54$) and an osteopathic practice ($n = 55$). Their primary

Table 14.1   Pain-provoking clinical tests used in the clinical examination; production of pain in back or leg constitutes a positive response (coded 1 = negative, 2 = positive)

Name	Description
PSOAS	Passive resisted hip flexion (knee bent) with patient sitting
FEMBAK	Passive flexion of both knees with patient prone
TENDER	Mid-line or paraspinal tenderness on moderate digital pressure (prone)
SLR	Passive straight leg raise (patient supine) – only positive at less than 50°
SLRQALT	Passive ankle dorsiflexion and medial hip rotation just below the point of pain on SLR
NOSITUP	Active attempt to sit up from supine with knees and hips flexed
FLXADD	Passive flexion-adduction of hip (supine)

complaint was of back and/or lower extremity symptoms attributable to lumbar dysfunction, and they were admitted to this study sequentially. Those with inflammatory, neoplastic and metabolic disorders were ineligible.

In addition to routine screening procedures, all the patients were examined by a single investigator (AKB) according to a structured protocol. This comprised a battery of seven pain-provoking clinical tests (PPCTs). The PPCTs, which previously have been shown to have individual relationships with symptomatic outcome (Burton & Getty, 1989), are detailed in Table 14.1. The patients were also asked to complete a pain-drawing, from which their site of symptoms was crudely determined as BAK (symptoms confined to low back and buttocks), or LEG (symptoms extending into one or both lower extremities), see Figure 14.1. Follow-up was by self-administered questionnaires, completed at 3 months

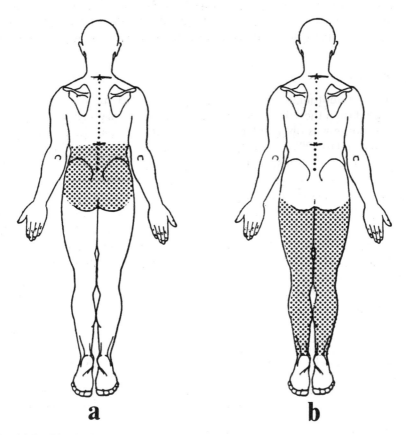

a   **b**

Fig. 14.1 The body-outlines used for the pain drawings; symptoms indicated in the shaded areas were classified as: (a) BAK or (b) LEG

and 1 year following consultation, from which forced-choice checklists enabled the symptomatic state to be recorded as either 'symptom-free' or 'persisting-symptoms'.

Statistical analysis was by means of discriminant analysis provided by the SPSS^x Information Analysis System (USA). The concept underlying this technique is that linear combinations (discriminant classification functions) of a set of predictor variables are formed and serve as the basis for classifying cases into one of a number of groups, i.e. a rule is derived from cases whose group membership is known, which can be used for allocating subjects for whom the group is unknown. In this study the discriminant functions were derived (using all nine variables as predictors) from 109 subjects for the 3-month assessment and from 89 subjects for the 1-year assessment, and the resulting classification from the analysis was compared with the actual distribution. This procedure gives satisfactory results with dichotomous as well as continuous variables (Norusis, 1986). In discriminant analysis the emphasis is on analysing the predictor variables simultaneously, thus providing important information about their relationships.

14.3 Results

The actual symptomatic state of the patients at 3 months and 1 year, determined from the self-assessment questionnaires, is given in Table 14.2: 100% response was obtained at 3 months, but at 1 year the proportion of responders fell to 82%. At the first assessment a little over half the patients had persisting symptoms, and at the 1-year point a similar number (representing 70% of responders) were suffering symptoms.

Table 14.3 shows the classification results from the discriminant analysis in respect of symptomatic state at the two assessment points. The column headed 'Actual Group' gives the known proportion in each group, whilst the 'Predicted Group' columns give the proportional classification resulting from use of the discriminant coefficients. The emboldened figure is the proportion-by-row correctly classified. At both assessment points those with 'persisting-symptoms' were better predicted (74 and 94%, respectively).

Table 14.2 Symptomatic outcome at 3 months and 1 year for 109 LBT patients, determined from self-assessment questionnaires. The numbers of patients are in parentheses

	Symptom-free	Persisting symptoms
3 months (109)	44% (48)	56% (61)
1 year (89)	30% (27)	70% (62)

Table 14.3 Classification results from discriminant analysis using nine variables (see text) as predictors of outcome at 3 months and 1 year. The numbers of patients are in parentheses

	Acutal group	Predicted group	
		Symptom-free	Persisting symptoms
3 months (109):			
Symptom-free	44% (48)	**56%** (27)	44% (21)
Persisting symptoms	56% (61)	26% (16)	**74%** (45)
1 year (89):			
Symptom-free	30% (27)	**30%** (8)	70% (19)
Persisting symptoms	70% (62)	7% (4)	**94%** (58)

Table 14.4 Accuracy of classification resulting from discriminant analysis based on data from Table 14.3, showing the proportions of predicted group membership which were correct

Predicted group	Symptom-free	Persisting symptoms
3 months	63%	68%
1 year	67%	75%

An alternative way to view these results is to express them in terms of the proportion of each predicted group being correctly classified, as opposed to the proportion of each actual group. Table 14.4 shows that around two-thirds of patients predicted as 'symptom-free' were indeed so, and that 'persisting-symptoms' at 3 months showed a similar level of accuracy; at 1 year the proportion of those predicted as 'persisting-symptoms' achieved an accuracy of 75%.

Whilst it is stressed that allocation of an individual case to a particular group depends on its values for all nine variables, it is possible, by looking at standardised coefficients, to obtain some idea of features which tend to influence the classification groupings. These standardised coefficients are given in Table 14.5, as are the discriminant function coefficients at group means. The discriminant function coefficients were negative for the 'symptom-free' group and positive for the 'persisting symptoms' group at each assessment.

Thus a positive response to a test (a higher variable value) will influence the classification of a case towards a 'symptom-free' grouping for variables with a negative coefficient, and towards a 'persisting symptoms' grouping for variables with a positive coefficient. In this light, one can suggest that a positive response to the SLR, BAK, FLXADD and FEMBAK tests were indicative of persisting symptoms at both assessments, and that LEG and

Table 14.5   Standardised canonical discriminant function coefficients produced by
discriminant analysis using nine variables, together with discriminant functions
evaluated at group means. Function is the discriminant function evaluated at group
means, derived from coefficients. Thus, high values (i.e. positive response) for
variables with a positive coefficient will contribute to allocation of a case as
'persisting-symptoms'. High values for variables with a negative coefficient will
contribute to allocation of a case as 'symptom-free'

| | 3 months | | 1 year | |
Variable	Coefficient	Variable	Coefficient
SLR	0.75	SLR	0.64
BAK	0.45	BAK	0.50
FLXADD	0.44	LEG	0.33
FEMBAK	0.23	NOSITUP	0.26
SLRQALT	−0.06	FEMBAK	0.23
LEG	−0.16	FLXADD	0.09
NOSITUP	−0.19	PSOAS	−0.54
PSOAS	−0.23	TENDER	−0.53
TENDER	−0.25	SLRQALT	−0.18
	Function		
Symptom-free	−0.49	Symptom-free	−0.71
Persisting symps	0.39	Persisting symps	0.31

NOSITUP further contributed at 1 year. However, it must be remembered
that a small number of positive responses among these variables could well
be countered by positive responses to the other tests, resulting in the case
being classified as symptom-free.

14.4 Discussion

The use of pain-provoking clinical tests (PPCTs) is part of most routine
clinical examination protocols for LBT patients, though their reliability has
been questioned (Nelson *et al.*, 1979). The PPCTs used here were largely
selected from literature reports showing good repeatability; however
consistency of interpretation when they are considered individually was not
necessarily shown in these reports. The straight leg raising test was
measured with a goniometer according to the repeatable protocol
described by Breig & Troup (1979), whilst the qualifying tests for root
tension (ankle dorsiflexion and medial hip rotation) were performed
independently, as recommended by Troup (1981). Lloyd & Troup (1983)
have shown good repeatability and predictive value for three of the other
tests used here (NOSITUP, PSOAS, FEMBAK). Passive flexion/adduc-
tion of the hip (FLXADD) has been described as a test for implicating the
sacro-iliac joint as the source of symptoms (Blower & Griffin, 1984), whilst

paraspinal tenderness is a universally used sign. Furthermore, the two pain descriptors (BAK and LEG) were deliberately kept simple to improve reliability (Waddell *et al.*, 1982).

Whilst some of the PPCTs had been shown to have some individual predictive value either for the clinical course of LBT or its recurrence, no previous report was found which considered their combined effect. A previous analysis of the data from the present subject population has shown that results from PPCTs contributed to the differentiation of patients attending hospital and office practice; the proposition was made that the two patient groups were dissimilar in ways that suggested that their complaints were of a different type (Burton & Getty, 1989). The present analysis has revealed that combinations of responses to this relatively small number of clinical tests (together with simple pain site descriptors) can identify a high proportion of LBT patients with a poor 3 month or 1 year prognosis.

It would seem, at least in the forseeable future, that clinicians (particularly those in office practice) will have to continue to rely on a clinical examination as a basis for classifying patients (identification of syndromes). In a climate of imprecise diagnosis, clinical classification might most usefully be based on the predictable outcome of the presenting spell. This study has demonstrated a means of identifying homogenous groups of patients (expressed in terms of two categories of outcome) from a simple clinical examination at the time of presentation. The power of this approach to classification may, in all probability, be improved by the inclusion of other variables such as psychological factors, which have previously been shown to be associated with outcome (Beals & Hickman, 1972; Burton & Getty, 1989).

In conclusion, although the model derived here can only be said to be applicable to this patient sample, it is suggested that suitably validated models could eventually be incorporated into the expert systems currently under development for clinical use (e.g. Gardner *et al.*, 1986).

References

Anderson, J. A. D. (1977). Problems of classification of low back pain, *Rheumatology and Rehabilitation*, **16**, 34–6.

Barker, M. E. (1977). Pain the back and leg – a general practice survey, *Rheumatology and Rehabilitation*, **16**, 37–45.

Beals, R. M. & Hickman, N. W. (1972). Industrial injuries of the back and extremities, *Journal of Bone and Joint Surgery*, **54A**, 1593–611.

Blower, P. W. & Griffin, A. J. (1984). Clinical sacroiliac tests in ankylosing spondylitis and other causes of low back pain – 2 studies. *Annals of the Rheumatic Diseases*, **43**, 192–5.

Breig, A. & Troup, J. D. G. (1979). Biomechanical considerations in the straight-leg-raise test, *Spine*, **4**, 242–50.

Burton, A. K. & Getty, C. J. M. (1989). Differences between 'orthopaedic' and 'osteopathic' patients with low back trouble. In: *Back pain: New approaches.* eds. M. Roland & J. R. Jenner. Manchester University Press, Manchester.

Gardner, A. D. H., Pursell, L. M., Murty, K. & Smith, D. G. (1986). The management of the clinical problem of spinal pain with the assistance of a microcomputer. In: *Back Pain, Methods for clinical investigation and assessment,* eds. D. W. L. Hukins & R. C. Mulholland, pp. 23–41. Manchester University Press, Manchester.

Heinrich, I., O'Hare, H., Sweetman, B. J. & Anderson, J. A. D. (1985). Validation aspects of an empirically derived classification for 'non-specific' low back pain, *Statistician,* **34**, 215–30.

Horal, J. (1969). The clinical appearance of low back pain disorders in the city of Gothenburg, Sweden. Comparisons of incapacitated probands with matched controls, *Acta Orthoapedica Scandinavica,* Supplement 118.

Jayson, M. I. V. (1970). The problem of backache, *The Practitioner,* **205**, 615–21.

Kersley, G. D., Collins, C. E., Dixon, A. St J., Jayson, M. I. V. & Jones, E. E. (1978). A search for evidence of clustering in 268 patients with non-specific back pain, *Annals of the Rheumatic Diseases,* **37**, 491.

Lankhorst, G. J., Van de Stadt, R. J., Vogelhaar, T. W., Van der Karst, J. R. & Prevo, A. J. H. (1982) Objectivity and repeatability of measurements in low back pain, *Scandinavian Journal of Rehabilitation Medicine,* **14**, 21–6.

La Rocca, H. & MacNab. I. (1969). Value of pre-employment radiographic assessment of the lumbar spine, *Canadian Medical Association Journal,* **101**, 49–54.

Lloyd, D. C. E. F. & Troup, J. D. G. (1983). Recurrent back pain and its prediction, *Journal of the Society of Occupational Medicine,* **33**, 66–74.

McQuaid Korenko, P., Boumphry, F., Hardy, R. W. & Sengstock, S. (1984). The efficacy of a back triage system – a prospective study. *International Society for the Study of the Lumbar Spine,* Toronto, June 1984.

Mathews, J. A., Mills, S. B., Jenkins, V. M., Grimes, S. M., Markel, M. J., Mathews, W., Scott, C. M. & Sittampalam, Y. (1983). Back pain and sciatica, four controlled trials, *British Association of Rheumatology and Rehabilitation, Annual Meeting 1983.*

Nachemson, A. & Andersson, G. B. J. (1982). Classification of low back pain, *Scandinavian Journal of Work and Environmental Health,* **8**, 134–6.

Nelson, M. A. (1986). The identification of back pain syndromes. In *Back Pain: Methods for clinical investigation and assessment,* eds. D. W. L. Hukins & R. C. Mulholland, pp. 13–15. Manchester University Press, Manchester.

Nelson, M. A., Allen, P., Clamp, S. E. & de Dombal, F. T. (1979). Reliability and reproducibility of clinical findings in low back pain *Spine,* **4**, 97–101.

Norusis, M. J. (1986). *SPSS Guide to Data Analysis,* SPSS Inc., Chicago.

Troup, J. D. G. (1981). Straight-leg-raising and the qualifying tests for increased root tension, *Spine,* **6**, 526–7.

Troup, J. D. G., Martin, J. W. & Lloyd, D. C. E. F. (1981). Back pain in industry. A prospective survey, *Spine,* **6**, 61–6.

Waddell, G., Main, C. J., Morris, C. W., Venner, R. M., Rae, P. S., Sharmy, S. H. & Golloway, H. (1982). Normality and reliability in the clinical assessment of backache, *British Medical Journal,* **284**, 1519–23.

Weber, H. & Burton, K. (1986). Rational treatment of low back trouble? *Clinical Biomechanics,* **1**, 160–7.

Wiltse, L., Newman, P. H. & Macnab, I. (1976). Classification of spondylolysis and spondylolysthesis, *Clinical Orthopaedics and Related Research,* **117**, 23–9.

Discussion

Fairbank: How many pain-provoking tests did you use?

Burton (in reply): Seven. We chose them not because we believed in them especially, but because either they were previously validated or because they were particularly suitable tests that had been reported by other people.

Fairbank: You recorded the presence and absence of pain?

Burton (in reply): Yes.

Fairbank: You were not too worried where they felt the pain?

Burton (in reply): Yes and no. Yes because most of the tests indicate where the patient has the pain.

Fairbank: Presumably if they had a pain on top of their head, that would not count.

Burton (in reply): That would not actually count, no.

Fairbank: What I am pursuing here is that when we looked at the reliability of physical examination, one of the most reliable tests was the pain induction test. It is a good sign both in terms of reliability and repeatability and is therefore quite a useful test.

McCoombe, P. F., Fairbank, J. C. T., Cockersole, B. C., & Pynsent, P. B. (1989). Reproducibility of physical signs in low back pain, *Spine*, **14**, 908–18.

Burton (in reply): That certainly applied in the tests we used. Previous descriptions of the tests tell you where the pain should be felt. For example, in flexion/adduction of the hip, which is supposedly a test for sacro-iliac dysfunction, you get a pain over the sacro-iliac joint if the test is positive. The prone-knee flexion test gives pain in the lower back, presumably due to passive extension of the lumbar spine. All the tests have some positive pain production in relevant areas and have been described elsewhere.

Mulholland: Was there a relationship between how many of the tests were positive? For example, would you say that if only two were positive, then they were less likely to have a poor prognosis, or was there any particular pain-provocation test which was particularly sensitive in predicticting prognosis? I would anticipate, for example, that a patient who had a major disc protrusion who has a lot of pain on straight leg raising would do worse than someone who had pain only if they bent forward.

Burton (in reply): The statistical technique does not work the way you want it to. We cannot pluck out individual variables that in themselves are more important. All we can do is get some idea of which direction each variable might tend to force people, but I do stress that the classification of any patient based on an analysis like this depends on their values for all variables. I am interested in what you said about your feeling that somebody would have a very poor 1-year prognosis if they had a very limited straight leg raising. I am not sure that that is true because one of the other variables we included was the qualifying tests for nerve root tension, and in fact a positive response to that variable contributed some decreased risk of chronicity. So it is almost as though one is floating around on a surface which is influenced by all these different factors and they are each pushing you in different directions.

Main: I wonder whether it might be relevant to share with you some results of a recent study we have done. We looked at general predictions of outcome of whether patients are symptomatic or not 1–2 years after they were first seen with back pain. You may or may not be surprised to know that the single best predictor is the level of distress they have initially. Factors such as straight leg raising had nothing to do with it. I just wondered whether you had either any demographic or psychosocial information about these patients, because what you may be picking up is people who become sensitised to pain in the first instance in the response to these tests. Any thoughts on that?

Burton (in reply): You have jumped a bit ahead of us. This is the first of a couple of papers. The second one will be presented at some other time. We have extended the variable set which does include pain drawings and inappropriate illness behaviour and what you are saying is, to a certain extent, what we found, that the psychosocial variables do have a considerable influence on the assessments after a year. Our intention in this study was to see whether simple clinical signs could produce a useful predictive model. Our conclusion is still that there is some room for clinical signs.

Main: I was not criticising what you had done, it was very interesting.

Fairbank (to Dr Main): Are your patients selected? We know that you have a particular interest and we have all seen the problems today for all of us in selection bias.

Main (in reply): The patients are routine referrals from GPs and orthopaedic surgeons. More likely the ones you normally see than the ones I normally talk about.

Burton: A year ago we gave a paper to the Society which showed that patients attending osteopaths, for instance, are different from the ones that attend orthopaedic surgeons. And working in a hospital, it seems likely from our experience that you are going to see the more chronic problems than the ones that have been dealt with at primary care level.

Burton, A. K. & Getty, C. J. M. (1989). Differences between 'orthopaedic' and 'osteopathic' patients with low back trouble. *Back pain: new approaches*. ed. M. Roland & J. R. Jenner. Manchester University Press, Manchester.

Deans: Can I ask how the predictions were tested? Are the percentages you quote from the same 109 used for the model?

Burton (in reply): Yes, the model is formulated from those whose outcome is already known.

Deans: You have not done any tests from a new unseen group?

Burton (in reply): No. that is the next step to see whether the model may be reproducible in the population. We are certainly not claiming that now.

15 *S. Simpson*

Evaluation of a technique for measuring lumbar lordosis in the clinical assessment of low back pain

15.1 Summary

This preliminary study was designed to evaluate a possible technique for the clinical measurement of spinal mobility and range of movement using a flexible ruler; 31 manual workers employed by British Steel suffering from low back pain were examined using this technique. The results were compared with those obtained from a matching group of workers who did not suffer from low back pain. The technique proved to be simple, accurate and highly reproducible as a clinical tool in the measurement of spinal mobility. A comparison of the observed spinal profile measurements demonstrated a significant difference in lumbar lordosis between the two groups. This suggested that the previously under-rated clinical sign of loss of lumbar lordosis might provide a useful measurement in evaluation of occupational low back pain. Other findings were that low back pain was associated with a decrease in extension measurements. There was also a correlation between height and the low back pain group. The study also highlighted further areas of investigation which might increase knowledge of the prediction and treatment of low back pain.

15.2 Screening methods to identify potential low back pain subjects

(1) *Clinical assessment*: A previous history of back or sciatic pain is one of the most reliable prognostic indicators.

(2) *Strength testing*: This is commonly used in the United States and some Scandinavian countries. Chronic low back pain is frequently accompanied by generalised weakness of the trunk muscles.

(3) *Measurement of lumbar spinal canal diameter*: The lumbar spinal canal diameter can be measured accurately by ultrasonic scanning.

Subjects with narrow canals are more likely to develop low back pain and incur sickness absence.

(4) *Radiological screening*: The value of radiological screening is controversial. The current consensus is that routine spinal X-rays are not cost or risk-benefit effective.

(5) *Spinal mobility*: Many different methods of assessing spinal mobility have been evaluated. They include radiographic techniques, goniometer studies, skin distraction methods, and flexible ruler measurements.

15.3 Design of study

15.3.1 *Hypothesis*
Spinal profile contours can be accurately measured using a flexicurve, as can spinal extension. The differences in readings obtained from subjects with low back pain and subjects without symptoms (controls) can be used as a practical way to quantify the degree of disability, and to monitor progress in an individual. It is possible that spinal profile measurements in asymptomatic individuals may identify those who have greatest risk of developing low back pain.

15.3.2 *Population and subject selection*
The study population consisted of all manual grade British Steel Corporation employees (8,000 men) based in Scotland. The subject group comprised men who were experiencing low back pain which radiated below the pelvis, and who had not been able to attend work for a period in excess of 4 weeks. Subjects who had undergone spinal surgery were excluded. Each employee has an individual attendance record. Information from self-certification or National Insurance Certificates is entered on this card. This information was used to identify the subject group. The pilot study lasted for 9 months, and during this time, 31 subjects satisfied the protocol definitions.

The control group consisted of men who were randomly selected whilst attending a clinic for reasons other than low back pain. They had never been away from work for more than 4 weeks with back pain, and were not currently suffering back pain. Employees were not further subdivided according to their individual jobs. The steel industry in Great Britain has undergone a major transformation in recent years with the loss of thousands of jobs. There are no 'light' jobs, and all require a reasonable degree of mobility.

15.4 **Technique of measurement**

Spinal profile and range of movement measurements were obtained by using a draughtsman's flexible curve. There are many different models available and they can be purchased from most stationary stores. Any are suitable as long as they are capable of bending in one plane, and maintain their shape. The flexicurve used in this study was obtained from a high street stationary store. It was marked at the centre, and at points 10 cm either side of the central mark. The length between the two extreme points was the measuring range (Figure 15.1).

Each subject was invited to attend for medical consultation, which comprised a full medical history and orthodox spinal examination. The subject was asked to stand in a comfortable position with feet together and arms hanging loosely by the side. No support was allowed. The subject was asked to look straight ahead. The lumbar lordosis was examined and the flexicurve was applied to the lumbar spine in the mid-line so that the central mark overlay the apex of the lumbar curve. The flexicurve was then moulded to the spinal contour (Figure 15.2) and the curve between the two extreme points traced onto graph paper.

The central point was aligned with a marked cross on the graph paper, and the outline of the curve traced. These readings were repeated twice.

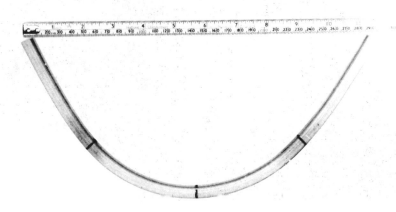

Fig. 15.1 The draughtsman's flexible curve

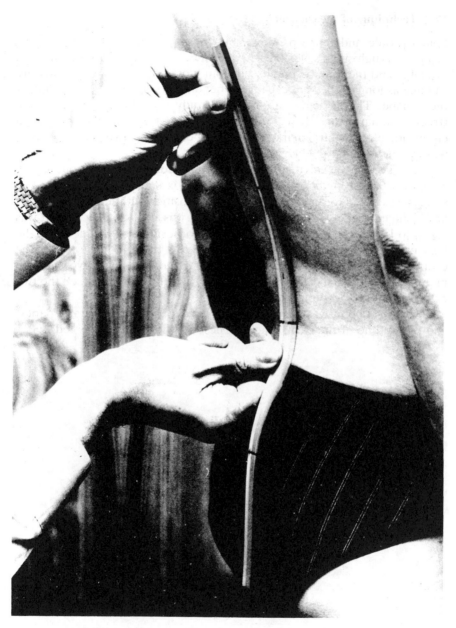

Fig. 15.2   Measurement of the standing profile

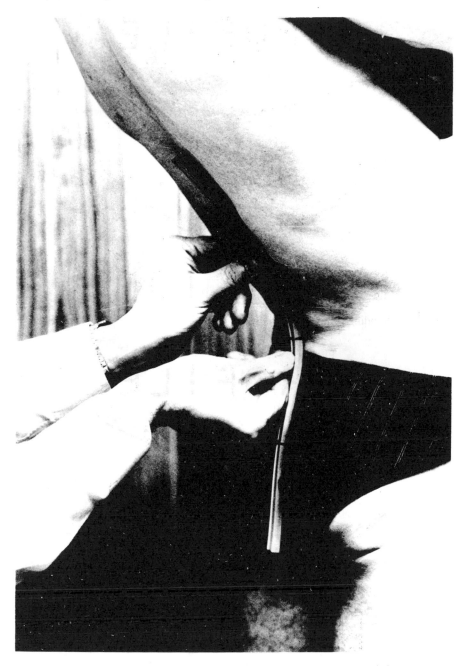

Fig. 15.3　Measurement of extension

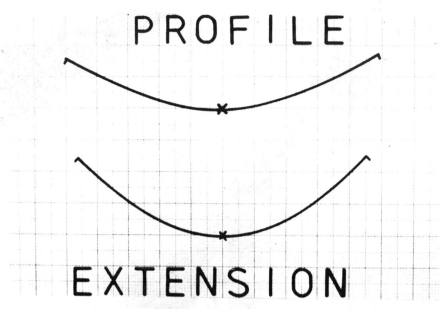

Fig. 15.4   Standing profile and extension curves

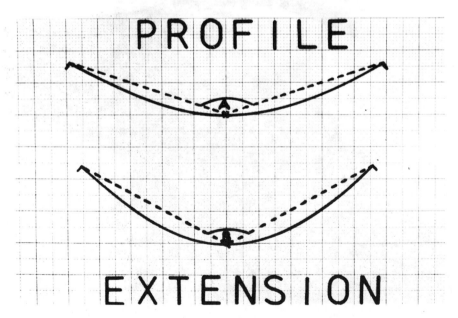

Fig. 15.5   Calculation of profile and extension measurements

The subject was then asked to bend backwards as far as he could without incurring pain. Three more profiles were then taken and these were called the extension measurements (Figure 15.3). They were also transferred to graph paper.

The tracings were then studied. A point was marked at each end of the profile which was the mid-point of the three recordings (Figure 15.4). A straight line was then drawn from the central mark to each of these two points. The angle between these two lines was measured at the central mark with a protractor. This angle (A) was called the lumbar angle and was measured in degrees (Figure 15.5). The same procedure was adopted for the extension measurement (B).

15.5 Results

The difference between the two angles gave the extension angle, measured in degrees. The differences between the profile measurements of the two groups can be seen in Figure 15.6.

The histograms were markedly different in shape, and analysis confirmed that these differences were statistically significant ($p < 0.002$). The low back pain subjects had flat backs with loss of the normal lumbar lordosis. Histograms were also drawn comparing extension measurements in the two groups (Figure 15.7). The histograms for the extension measurements of the two groups were even more marked. The differences were statistically significant ($p < 0.00001$).

There was also a statistically significant relationship between height and

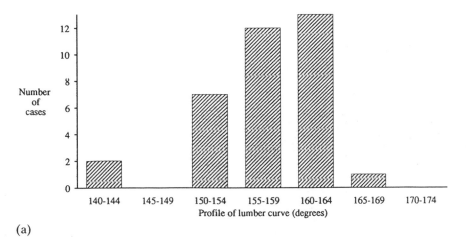

(a)

Fig. 15.6 (a, above) Control profiles; (b, overleaf) subject profiles

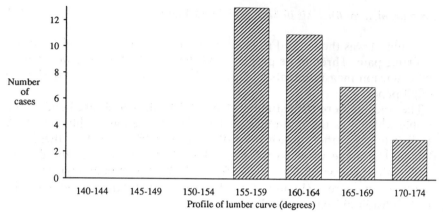

Fig. 15.6(b)

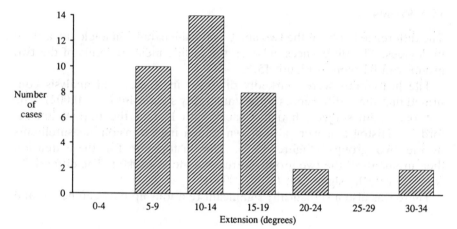

Fig. 15.7(a)

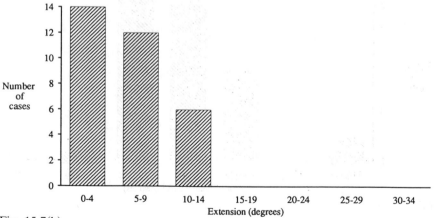

Fig. 15.7(b)

Fig. 15.7   (a) Control extensions; (b) subject extensions

Table 15.1   Weight and height (means ± SD)

	Height (m)	Weight (kg)
Subjects	1.78 ± 0.06	79.7 ± 13.1
Controls	1.72 ± 0.06	76.5 ± 8.86

the subject group suffering from low back pain ($p < 0.01$) Weight was not related to either group (Table 15.1). The results may be summarised as;

(1)   the average profile was different in the two groups;

(2)   the average extension was different in the two groups;

(3)   extension decline was not associated with age in either group;

(4)   there was a relationship between height and the subject group who suffered from low back pain, weight was not associated with either group;

(5)   age had no association with profile in either group.

15.6 Conclusion

The spinal profile was readily and accurately measurable. Although a shallow curve was significantly related to the presence of low back pain there were many cases which overlapped. For example, controls without back pain and with a shallow back, and *vice versa*. Hence the value of the spinal profile as a screening tool is limited. However, it does provide a tool for the objective measurements of the severity of the low back pain which is independent of the patient's description of his symptoms and do not depend on his cooperation during the examination.

It is possible that the spinal contour may itself be of predictive value in asymptomatic individuals. This could only be established in a large prospective screening study. It would also be intriguing to know whether profile measurements taken at the beginning of an episode of low back pain would have any prognositic significance. This could also only be ascertained by a prospective study.

Spinal profile measurements were obtained which suggested that the degree of lumbar lordosis was an important and previously under-rated clinical sign. It was also established that individuals with low back pain had measurable reductions in extension movements. In this study of 31 patients, height was identified as a risk factor.

The problems posed by low back pain surely concerns every occupational physician. As controversy surrounds the merits of may treatments for low back pain, any addition to the range of objective measuring devices is of value.

Acknowledgements

I would like to express my gratitude to Dr R. Knill-Jones and the statisticians of the Department of Community Medicine, University of Glasgow, for their help in the analysis of the data. I am grateful to Dr A. Sinclair (Chief Medical Officer, British Steel Corporation) for his advice and permission to publish these results. I am especially appreciative of the constant help and encouragement I received from Dr G. Sharp (Consulting Occupational Physician, Forth Valley Health Board).

Discussion

Barker: You say you put the marker at the apex of the curve of the lumbar spine, but if these patients have got flat lumbar spines, how did you manage to decide where the apex was?

Simpson (in reply): It was occasionally difficult, but when somebody has a 'flat back', there is always a degree of curve and you can eyeball where you think the centre of this curve is. That was a weakness of the study which was recognised. I did get a number of people to look at different subjects and say where they thought the apex would be. We all agreed within a certain distance. Even deliberately choosing a mark one or two centimetres away from where you felt the apex was did not affect the results, so the exact localisation did not appear to be crucially important.

Eisenstein: Did you measure forward bending or observe forward bending, perhaps during a clinical examination, on these same patients? If you did were you puzzled perhaps by a group of patients who appeared to have almost no backward bending with your measure, but could touch their toes on forward bending?

Simpson (in reply): Yes, that is a very good question. I was going to include flexion movements in this study but I discovered exactly what you found. We have all seen patients with back pain who can bend over and touch their toes, and if you examine this movement it seems to come from the hip rather than the back.

Frank: The objective method of lumbar spine flexion is, if I remember correctly, to find L5 and you go 10 cm above and 5 cm below (it is all written up by Macrae and White years ago) that gives you objective spinal movement, nothing to do with hip flexion at all. So you can get around that problem.

Macrae I. F. & Wright, V. (1969). Measurement of back movement, *Annals of Rheumatic Disease*, **28**, 584–9.

Simpson (in reply): The flexicurve technique does that as well.

Frank: Yes, I know. I am just commenting and I do not think we should get distracted from that.

Porter: Were the controls matched for age?

Simpson (in reply): Yes they were. There were 31 subjects who satisfied the protocol definitions and I divided them into eight bands of 5 years. I took as my controls people who were attending for health screening or vaccinations or anything unconnected with low back pain. If I had six people aged 36–40, I made sure I had six controls in the same age range. At the end of the study it got to the stage where I was saying to the nurses, 'Any 59 year olds who come in who have not got back pain, let me know.'

Porter: Was the time of day controlled?

Simpson (in reply): It was controlled in as much as it was by the hours that I was working. I did not think of that as an important factor.

Mitchell: In any new technique, especially a clinically related one, it is essential to know something about acceptable degrees of reproducibility. Would you care to comment on inter-observer variations in your study?

Simpson (in reply): As far as the intra-observer technique was concerned, we found that the angles could be reproduced within a degree or two. The physiotherapist and three nurses who were working in the department all took measurements from one individual who did not have back pain, and their results were studied to assess inter-observer error. The range of measurement was five degrees between the lowest and highest figure. Extension measurements varied by only one degree. I am not sure why this measurement should be the most consistent.

McDonald: Speaking from a viewpoint of thinking that increased lumbar lordosis is the most common symptomatic postural fault, I look rather critically at what you produce. Firstly, having people who have an unusually flat back and restricted extension as a group who run into problems does not mean that there is not also another group of people who go to the opposite extreme of having excess lumbar lordosis who run into symptoms. The other point about it is that you produced one measurement of lumbar lordosis. I think that there is a group of people who extend their thoracic kyphosis right down into the lumbar region, right down into L3 or L4, and then have rather an acute little lordosis right at the base of the spine where those lower joints seem to be hyperextended and by closing the posterior compartment produce symptoms. Your measurement would not really differentiate those people who presumably have a flat back from their middle to upper lumbar spine but would actually be suffering hyperlordotic problems at the extreme lumbosacral junction.

Simpson (in reply): The first point you made, if I understood you correctly, was that there are individuals with increased lumbar lordosis and increased mobility who have low back pain. I am aware of individuals like that, but I did not find any in this study. In my experience they are a minority problem.

Concerning the second point that you made, you do get a lot of extension in the thoracic region and it is difficult to separate that from lumbar movement. I did not go into this in my presentation but I did take anatomical land marks of all the lumbar vertebrae and the lower thoracic ones and calculated ranges of movement by drawing tangents, much in the way Kim Burton (1986) has described. Those results are very interesting but are also very difficult to interpret.

Burton A. K. (1986). Regional lumbar sagittal mobility; measurement by flexicurves. Clinical Biomechanics, **1**, 20.

Mulholland: These patients that had back pain, when you saw them, had a flat back. Did you feel that this was a response to their disability? Do you know if it reversed when their particular episode was over or do you suppose that the fact that they were suffering back pain was because they had flat backs? Many people teach that someone who has back pain will usually get better just by recovering their lumbar lordosis. Do you think that the flat back is due to their back pain or they were pre-exisiting abnormalities which made them have back pain?

Simpson (in reply): That is a very fundamental point. My own view is that if you have a back problem you then have a flat back. Now whether that is because of muscle spasm I am not sure. I have followed some of these patients up and I put these curves that I have taken onto transparencies and I can overlap them over a period of time. You find that once the patient says the pain is less then you find the movement is greater and the flat back does disappear. I am sure physiotherapists would agree that you have got to get this lower lumbar back curve right if you want to get better. If you get rid of the pain then this is possible.

Index